Exploring the Skills of Mental Health Nurses

HARRY GIJBELS
PHILIP BURNARD

Avebury

Aldershot • Brookfield USA • Hong Kong • Singapore • Sydney

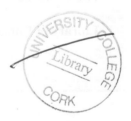

Published by
Avebury
Ashgate Publishing Limited
Gower House
Croft Road
Aldershot
Hants GU11 3HR
England

Ashgate Publishing Company
Old Post Road
Brookfield
Vermont 05036
USA

British Library Cataloguing in Publication Data

Gijbels, Harry
    Exploring the Skills of Mental Health Nurses
    I. Title II. Burnard, Philip
    610.7368
ISBN 1 85628 662 2

Library of Congress Catalog Card Number: 95-76421

Printed and bound in Great Britain by
Athenaeum Press Ltd, Gateshead, Tyne & Wear

Contents

Contents

1 Introduction and aims of the study

It could reasonably be assumed that mental health nursing is an obvious useful activity, in which mental health nurses are engaged on a daily basis in a variety of settings and with a wide range of client groups.

Over the last few decades however this activity has received, and still receives, a great deal of criticism. This relates to issues regarding the roles and skills of mental health nursing, the future direction of this profession, and the position and influence that nurses have in relation to other disciplines within mental health care provision.

Davis (1990) argues that mental health nursing research has established itself over the last twenty years. Reviewing the mental health nursing literature over a twenty year period, he identifies trends in research content and methodology (Davis 1981, 1986, 1990). Initially, studies were mainly attempts to define and evaluate the nurses' role, particularly in relation to communication and nurse-patient relationships. The early 1980's saw a shift towards educational issues, but increasingly two areas became more prominent, namely studies around community psychiatric nursing, and research into the nurse as therapist. Davis' (1990) last review saw a further proliferation of these two areas. He points out that most studies were of a descriptive nature, although there were some examples of action, comparative and experimental research.

Brooking (1985) observes that the concentration on these specialist areas is largely irrelevant to the work of most mental health nurses. Indeed, it has been argued that there is a need for research in those areas which demonstrates how the nursing action engaged in by the majority of mental health nurses in their day-to-day work can be of benefit to patients (Thomas 1992).

The largest proportion of mental health nurses - 80 000 - are employed in hospital units. Nearly 60 000 psychiatric in-patients places are remaining, of which 16 000 are in local hospital psychiatric units (O.H.E. 1989). Although a decline in the use of psychiatric hospitalisation has taken place, and a further decrease is anticipated, in-patient care, of as yet undetermined structure and format, is likely to remain as a back-up resource to be used when community services or facilities are inadequate or unavailable (Marks and Scott 1990).

It has been suggested that the vital role that mental health nurses perform in the traditional hospital based settings may be considered of less prestige, and therefore seems to be getting less attention (Keltner 1985). Indeed, research studies regarding the work of hospital based nurses appears to have taken a back seat since the studies undertaken in the 1970's and early 1980's (Altschul 1972; Cormack 1976, 1983; Towell 1975; Carr 1979). Keltner (1985) asserts that nurses in hospital settings suffer from role confusion and are in conflict about their practice and their worth. Although he refers the American context, similar concerns have been expressed in this country. The recent review of mental health nursing (D.O.H. 1994a) found that some nurses working within in-patient settings felt that their skills were undervalued, especially when compared with those working in community settings. This is not a new finding. Barker (1989), some years earlier, referred to an emerging class consciousness in nursing, and argues that the emphasis on community care has encouraged many hospital based nurses to feel like second class citizens. He wonders whether those working in the acute setting are the last bastion of generalists, beyond control to change. Smith (1988) suggests that nurses need to examine their job content.

She fears that if these nurses are not more judicious, they may find themselves on the outside looking in, while others - by which she presumably means other mental health professionals -get on with the "real" work. She fails to make explicit what this "real" work consists of.

It has been suggested that it is a truism that nursing is a skills based profession (Davis 1990). He believes that mental health nursing has a skills profile that is weighted towards interpersonal problem solving

2

and planning, emphasising however that it is the intelligent informed use of those skills.

The prescriptive mental health nursing literature identifies a range of skills that nurses should use (Reynolds and Cormack 1990; Brooking et al 1992; Wright and Giddey 1993). Equally, the Syllabus of Training (E.N.B. 1982) prescribes a skills based curriculum. It can then be assumed that mental health nursing skills are initially influenced by education.

Various authors have drawn attention to the discrepancies that exists between the prescribed and described role of mental health nursing in ward based settings (Cormack 1976, 1983; Carr 1979). Although they have attempted to explain these discrepancies, it seems that little is known about the perceptions that nurses have about their skills, what skills they value and employ, and what factors influence the use of their skills. Do they indeed use a wide variety of approaches and skills as identified in textbooks and in the 1982 E.N.B. syllabus, or can it be assumed that they may have an understanding of those approaches, but lack the necessary skills and opportunities to implement these?

Aims of the study

Ward based mental health nurses, who work in an acute psychiatric admission until attached to a district general hospital, are at the centre of this study. The focus is on the therapeutic skills that nurses use in that setting, and factors that may influence the way those skills are employed.

Within this focus, a number of aims have been identified. Firstly, to review the mental health nursing literature, with a view to explore contemporary issues in relation to the roles and skills of mental health nurses, and to examine the prescriptive and descriptive literature in relation to ward based mental health nursing practice. Secondly, to collect, through semi-structured interviews, information from nurses and other health professionals about their perceptions of mental health nursing skills. Thirdly, to analyse, describe and discuss this information, with a view to gain a better understanding of how nurses and other health professionals perceive these skills. Fourthly, to offer possible implications and recommendations on the basis of these findings.

The study then has a qualitative nature by using the semi-structured interview as a method of data collection, and by adopting the thematic content analysis as a method of data analysis. Adopting this emic approach, the author intends to provide an account of how nurses and other health professionals understand the skills of mental health nurses in an acute psychiatric admission environment.

2 The literature review

The purpose of this review is to provide a broad overview of the contemporary debate about the roles, the skills, and the position of mental health nursing, as documented both in the prescriptive and descriptive literature. To set this overview in context, a brief historical perspective will initially be offered.

An historical overview

Tracing the past may help to identify some factors that have led to contemporary mental health nursing practice. The history of mental health nursing suggests that it simply grew, without ever asking why and how (Barker 1990).

A number of authors have explored the history of mental health nursing, among them Barker (1990) and Nolan (1993). Nolan (1993) traces its development back to ancient Greece, where Seranus already seemed to be thinking about client centred approaches. He also points out that those eager to describe mental health nursing skills today would do well to consider writers who attempted to define the care of the mentally ill in the 16th and 17th century, in which three elements to successful care were considered: understanding, consent and compassion.

The formal concept of mental health nursing emerged initially from the patronage of the medical profession, and was later influenced by developments in psychology and sociology. Weir (1992) describes one of the earliest attempts - in the mid 19th century - at providing attendants with some form of training through a series of one off lectures. Formal training however dates back to 1891. Man Cheung Chung and Nolan (1994) argue that the introduction of this formal training did not lead to greater control for these attendants, but rather resulted in further subservience towards the medical profession. They claim that the positivistic tradition of the day has been a perverted force in its influence on the history of mental health care in this country, and subsequently mental health nursing training and practice.

The role of attendants during the late 19th and early 20th century has been described as "occupying the middle ground between doctors and patients" (Nolan 1993). He illustrates that these attendants came from varied backgrounds: strong men from a farm labouring background, disciplined ex-servicemen, and subservient ex-butlers. Their functions were those of rule keeper, servant, spiritual guide, and intermediary between "high status doctors and uncivilised patients". Contemporary research, for example by Cormack (1976, 1983), who examined the role of the mental health nurse, suggests that the words may have changed, but not the actions.

The early part of the 20th century saw little change, with a workforce deeply entrenched in routine, institutionalised practices, while innovative community services were being developed, in which nurses were not involved.

Nolan (1993) suggests that the Second World War provided nurses with opportunities to acquire skills, that they would never have acquired during their training, mainly influenced by the thinking of people like Dr Maxwell Jones and Dr Main, who were instrumental in the development of innovative approaches, based on the principles of the therapeutic community.

During the last 40 years the development of mental health nursing has been influenced by developments in psychopharmacology, changes in social policy, such as the shift towards community oriented services, the arrival of other mental health workers, such as social workers and occupational therapists, educational innovations, such as the 1982 ENB syllabus, but also the demise of local Schools of Nursing, and developments in nursing research. Nolan (1993) argues that on the basis of historical evidence, nurses should now feel empowered to disown the historical stereotypes with which they have been unfairly labelled, and to begin to reconstruct their past without fear. Similar thoughts are expressed by Hopton (1993), who supports the idea of a critical re-evaluation of the history of mental health nursing.

The contemporary debate

The recent debate about mental health nursing seems to indicate confusion and conflict over its role and its sense of direction. Burnard (1990) claims that mental health nursing is in "something of a wilderness" and argues that "we do not really know what good psychiatric nursing is" (p.20). It seems that not only do we not know what good psychiatric nursing is, we appear to still find it difficult to define what psychiatric nursing per se is. The review of mental health nursing (D.O.H. 1994a) found that some practitioners struggled with the task of defining mental health nursing, and took, not surprisingly one might add, a profession specific rather than a user focused perspective. Another indication of the difficulty of defining mental health nursing is illustrated in a recent report by the Audit Commission (1994). This report included a glossary of the key professionals in mental health care. The roles of these professionals was briefly described. However, under the heading "psychiatric nurses" it reads:

> 'are the most numerous professionals in mental health. Most of their basic training takes place in hospital...'

without any reference to their role.

The concept of mental health nursing remains insecure and hazy, asserts Barker (1990), functioning mainly as a medical support system, although he points out that it has become common practice to assert the interpersonal basis of mental health nursing, influenced by for example the theories of Peplau (1952) and Rogers (1951). Indeed, some argue that a shift has taken place from a medical to a psycho-social orientation (Adams 1991; Butterworth 1987). Adams (1991) even makes the claim that mental health nursing now embraces a holistic paradigm, suggesting - arguably - the existence of a mental health nursing paradigm. Lacey (1993) however points out that psychiatric nursing practice is mainly based on borrowed theories which have not led to a distinct psychiatric nursing approach. This is, in some way, recognised by the report of the mental health nursing review (D.O.H. 1994a), that indicates that it is difficult to lay exclusive claim to the possession of mental health nursing skills, as other professional groups also operate from related skills and knowledge bases. The report however suggests that it is the combination of these particular skills, linked with values and practices common to the nursing profession as a whole, which provides the unique expertise of mental health nursing. The therapeutic use of self and the client centred philosophy is highlighted as the core and focus of this expertise. Barker (1994) welcomes this reinforcement of the "human core" of mental health nursing.

For others however the image of interpersonal relationships in mental health nursing is more a matter of professional aspiration than established fact (Isles 1986).

Altschul (1984) suggests that in the past mental health nursing could be clearly identified, because of its close association with the medical model. She argues that if this association is abandoned, then "all the world becomes the object of psychiatric nursing practice", which may create difficulties in differentiating psychiatric nursing practice from the practice of others:

> "good practice in psychiatric nursing must imply that it is nurses who are doing something and that this practice is in some way different from that of other people and specific to nurses" (Altschul 1984:37).

Altschul (1984) supports her argument by stating that if the sick-role is denied to the patient, then the justification for having nurses may have vanished too. It could be argued that she thereby denies the potential for nurses to be engaged in the prevention of mental ill-health and the promotion of mental health. Although her argument seems to imply that the recipient of care determines the boundaries of practice, she also makes a case for defining mental health nursing practice simply by identifying what nurses do. In other words: mental health nursing is what mental health nursing does.

Adding further confusion to the debate, she argues that she does not know what good practice is, nor by what criteria to judge this,

8

concluding that mental health nurses may not have to do anything, they merely have to be:

> "like a mother or a friend; it is what you might do, not what you are in fact doing" (Altschul 1984:38).

Several authors have attempted to conceptualise mental health nursing in a framework for practice, thereby providing it with a direction (Peplau 1952; Reed 1987; Kerr 1990). Peplau's (1952) interpersonal framework was referred to earlier. Reed (1987) observes that mental health nurses often adopt an eclectic approach to intervention, incorporating psycho-analytical, behavioural and humanistic theories. She proposes what seems to be a complicated framework, based on nursing's suggested metaparadigm of person, environment, health and nursing practice, incorporating the often opposing ideas put forward by nurse theorists during the last 25 years. Hopton (1993) comments that the adoption of haphazard eclecticism owes more to "common sense" assumptions that it does to serious enquiry. Kerr's (1990) ego competency model seems to be a more practical guide to practice, based on assessment of ego strengths and deficits. This appears to have a psychological rather than a nursing foundation.

The value of conceptual nursing frameworks for mental health nursing practice has as yet not been extensively demonstrated. Wardle and Mandle (1989) found that of the 27 nurses they interviewed, only 6 were able to articulate a conceptual model containing the concepts of person, environment, health and nursing. Over half the respondents described some of the concepts. It could be argued however that nurses are guided by conceptual frameworks that have been developed by other disciplines.

Whyte (1985) suggests that the confusion and conflict within mental health nursing may have their origin in nurses' inability to articulate what it is they do, how they do it, and what benefits are gained by their actions. It seems that theoretical or ideological discussions have not been a major preoccupation among mental health nurses, although a recent change has been suggested (White 1985). If mental health nursing is to survive, nurses themselves need to address these questions (Clarke 1988; Smith 1988), before others do it for them (Butterworth 1987).

Nursing as therapy or care

Much of the debate seems to concentrate on whether mental health nurses are therapists in their own right, or primarily guardians, assisting others in the delivery of therapeutic interventions. Cox (1990) proposes that this ambiguity stems from the ambiguity in psychiatry itself: the composite representation of the medical and interdisciplinary approach. Her arguably dubious contention is that within education there is an alignment with the latter, in which students are encouraged to define themselves as therapists, even though this view may not be shared or agreed upon by other members of the multi-disciplinary team. This may result in conflicting messages about the level of skill and involvement. Cox (1990), in an attempt to redefine the role, argues for the formal recognition of psychotherapy as a central nursing function.

Although Cox refers to the American context, a similar debate is developing in this country (Isles 1986; Vousden 1986; Farrington 1992). There are those who claim that their role is more to do with treatment than care and seek a close affiliation with other mental health professionals. Others believe that nursing, irrespective of the area of practice, has certain essential defining characteristics, with an emphasis on providing care, not treatment (Wilson Barnett 1988). Farrington (1992) argues that the latter may lead mental health nursing on the road to invisibility, supporting his argument with recent educational developments, such as Project 2000 with its common core emphasis.

Prescribed roles and skills

The previous section has highlighted the confusion in the role and position of the mental health nurse. Cormack's (1976, 1983) differentiation between what nurses do - the described role - and what nurses apparently ought to do - the prescribed role - seems a useful way to explore and maybe clarify this confusion. The focus, within the context of this study, will be on the roles and skills that nurses employ, or apparently should employ, in the area of acute mental health nursing practice.

Cormack (1983) divides the prescriptive role into three broad areas. The first identifies the nurse as the doctor's assistant, mediating between doctor and patient, but also performing medical expressive roles, such as administering medication. This role has its roots in the custodial tradition of mental health care. The second role, which has an administrative nature, is closely associated with this tradition. This role, according to Corwin (1961), has tended to be better rewarded, although it could be argued that the clinical grading exercise during the late 1980's was an attempt to value and reward the clinical role and skills of the nurse. The third role has a multi-dimensional character, encompassing a range of personal therapeutic roles, influenced by psychological and sociological treatment approaches, such as counselling, psychotherapy, sociotherapy and behaviour therapy.

This third role has received increased attention by those seeking to prescribe a role for mental health nurses which is relatively independent of other staff groups, and attempts to place mental health nurses in a formal, autonomous role. The 1982 ENB syllabus for example identifies the roles of therapist, counsellor, teacher and health educator. Cormack (1983) argues that the shift towards this therapeutic role was not based on a unilateral decision by mental health nurses, but resulted from a wider multi-disciplinary shift towards a therapeutic ideology. It is not clear how influential nurses themselves have been in the changing nature of their position.

This therapeutic potential of mental health nurses has been proposed for the last 25 years, although the research evidence is still missing (Barker 1990). He asserts that at present no commonly accepted definition appears to exist in mental health nursing as to what this potential may consist of.

In the absence of any central directives, and recognising the importance of a definitive statement, the Joint Committee of Mental Health Nursing (1986) published a document, outlining the role of the mental health nurse. This document identifies the nurse as delivering, or helping to deliver, an extensive repertoire of therapeutic approaches, personally, or in co-ordination with the multi-disciplinary care team. This therapeutic potential continues to be prescribed and emphasised in textbooks as the primary role of mental health nurses (for example Reynolds and Cormack 1990). They argue that nurses employ strategies which are used to diagnose and personally influence patient responses. Their thinking seems influenced by the American Nurses' Association's (1980) claim, and implicitly for mental health nursing practice:

"the diagnosis and treatment of human responses to actual and potential health problems" (Reynolds and Cormack 1990:13).

Although this definition attempts a departure from the disease oriented approach, it only seems to recreate a different diagnostic framework. The vagueness of the definition makes it equally applicable to the work of other mental health professionals. Indeed, Brooking et al (1992) would welcome a blurring of role boundaries in so far as this results in the provision of more effective and efficient services for patients, arguing that psychiatrists do not have exclusive expertise to diagnose and treat, any more than nurses have the prerogative to caring.

Therapeutic skills

It has been suggested that the skills of mental health nurses "merit celebration" (Peplau 1987:29). She describes a skill as a co-ordinated pattern of mental and physical activity, and suggests that the most relevant skills for mental health nurses fall within the perceptual, intellectual and communicative categories, applied within the nurse-patient relationship. Peplau (1987) argues that, in some degrees, these skills are either lacking, undeveloped, misused or distorted in the recipients of care.

Peplau's (1987) description of a skill is broadened by that of Argyris and Schon (1976), who suggest that a skill is a dimension of ability in which one behaves effectively in situations of action. Skills, according to them, move along a continuum of ability and behaviour in a certain context. Within the context of mental health nursing, it seems open for debate what these "effective behaviours" and "dimensions of ability" are.

The development of skills in mental health nursing can be traced back to the custodial-companionship skills, to mothering skills, technical skills, skills related to socialising activities, health teaching, counselling skills, and a range of other treatment modalities, which have proliferated over the last few decades (Peplau 1984). She concludes that world-wide a shift is taking place towards therapeutic nursing. According to Sloboda (1993) there are five principal characteristics of activities that make up what is referred to as a skill: fluency, rapidity, automatically, simultaneity and knowledge. He suggests that it is not a matter of having knowledge per se, but having it available when required, at the appropriate time, in response to the situation that demands its use. Skilful behaviour is the result of motivation, belief and practice, and, Sloboda (1993) argues, having innate potential.

Therapeutic nursing is indeed receiving increased attention. Hockey (1991) suggests it has to do with those nursing activities which have a healing effect, or those which result in a movement towards health and wellness. A framework is offered by McMahon (1991), in which he identifies the following categories:

- developing partnership, intimacy, reciprocity in nurse-patient relationship.
- manipulating the environment.
- teaching.
- providing comfort.
- utilising tested physical interventions.
- adopting complementary health practices.

It could be argued that the addition of complementary health practices turns nursing into a therapeutic activity, assuming that the other activities are already perceived as part of a nurse's repertoire of skills. Hockey's (1991) notion seems equally vague. She does appear to imply that there is such a thing as non-therapeutic nursing, although it could be claimed that such an activity would not deserve the term "nursing" at all.

The therapeutic skills of the mental health nurse seem to have been influenced by a variety of theoretical perspectives, such as interpersonal, psychodynamic and humanistic influences. Altschul (1984) argues that the interpersonal approach may be beneficial for nurses, but wonders whether it is good for patients. Ending relationships may be determined not by mutual negotiation and achieved outcomes, but by factors such as the nurse's holidays or internal rotation. She also suggests that the principle underlying this approach may have to do, more, with providing cheap second rate therapy as a substitute for prestigious psychotherapy by psychiatrists.

Keltner (1985) thinks that nurses may struggle between the practice of therapy and the act of being therapeutic. He attempts to clarify these blurring concepts by offering a therapeutic continuum ranging from psychotherapeutic behaviour to psychotherapy. Respect, a desire to help, and understanding are identified as the minimum standard of therapeutic activities on this continuum. Providing structure and working from a theoretical therapeutic model then moves the nurse along the continuum to psychotherapeutic practice.

Being therapeutic however is not enough. Keltner (1985) argues for the nurse to be a therapeutic manager: managing psycho-pharmacology, psychopathology, the environment, and the therapeutic nurse-patient relationship. A rather all embracing task, which seems to suggest managerial activities, but excluding nurses from being involved in the practice of psychotherapy.

It has also been suggested that the therapeutic skills of nurses and psychotherapists are complementary. Bunch (1985) proposes that the difference lies in the nature and duration of contact: the nurse focuses on immediate needs, while the primary therapist focuses on underlying dynamic processes. Again, this appears to indicate that Bunch (1985) sees no role for nurses as therapeutic agents in their own right.

Keltner's (1985) continuum shows similarities to the structure that Brown and Pedder (1991) offer, which may help nurses identify at what level they function. They suggest that the first level requires an awareness of the person as well as the problem, which requires skills to communicate and emphathise. Roger's (1951) client-centred therapy is associated with this level. The second level, while containing elements of the first, adds the start of the therapeutic alliance. The third level focuses on the concepts of transference and countertransference within the therapeutic relationship.

It could be argued that these levels represent three different theoretical ideologies, rather than a continuum: client-centred therapy, supportive psychotherapy, and psycho-analytic therapy. The emphasis in all three however seems to be on affecting change through a therapeutic relationship.

Within mental health nursing however, it has been suggested that "no therapeutic system" seems to be the most common system practised (Barker 1989).

Peplau (1987) argues, without any support for her argument, that the crucial question now is: "What do nurses remedy?" instead of "What do nurses do?" implying that there is sufficient evidence about nurses' effectiveness in their employment of skills. Others are less optimistic about the skills of mental health nurses. Nolan (1993) wonders whether there is sufficient understanding as yet of what a skill is in relation to mental health care, and asks himself the question what a skilful nurse is. Equally, Burnard (1989) claims that the crux of the matter is that we still do not know what mental health nursing skills are, or what skills are therapeutic.

In 1982 the English National Board introduced a skills based syllabus for mental health nurse training (ENB 1982). This, the document claims, was justified for a number of reasons. Firstly, to give a clear statement of the skills of the mental health nurse, which includes intellectual, personal, interpersonal, practical and organisational skills. Secondly, this emphasis on skills identifies mental health nursing as essentially a human activity. Thirdly, to highlight self-awareness skills as vital for all therapeutic interaction.

The syllabus has not been without its critics. Nolan (1993) argues that the assumptions that mental health nursing is a skills based profession, that nursing competencies can be learned, and that the skills cited in the syllabus would enable patients to get better, were untested. Indeed, he asserts that no evidence was produced to indicate what patients found skilful in the behaviour of nurses.

Barker (1989) also criticises the syllabus for its emphasis on nursing skills, claiming that of the extensive list of 150 skills, he can only find about six which may have something to do with nursing. Unfortunately, he fails to identify these six for the reader. Barker (1989) wonders why they are called "nursing" skills, arguing that they may be learned by nurses, but that does not make them their property. This appears to reflect his notion that a body of expertise does not belong to any particular discipline. He concludes that the authors of the syllabus missed the opportunity to come clean about the bankrupt state of mental health nursing, by ignoring to acknowledge "the wilderness location of mental health nursing":

> "if we are to teach only interventions which have been defined, researched and found to be effective, then it will be an exceptionally short module of skills training indeed". (Barker 1989:24).

Barber (1986) on the other hand welcomes the syllabus, but suggests it arrived too late, claiming that other mental health professionals had already filled the gaps, such as facilitating group work. He does however favour the emphasis on skills based on humanistic psychology, suggesting that nurses should become experts in counselling and group work.

Described roles and skills

Having explored the roles and skills that hospital based mental health nurses are assumed to perform, in this section the author reviews the descriptive literature in relation to the roles and skills that nurses apparently carry out in practice. The emphasis will be on those studies, published since the early 1970's, that relate to the area under study, and will therefore exclude specialist hospital based units, such as forensic psychiatric units and child and adolescent psychiatric units.

Studies into hospital based mental health nursing have been scarce during the last 25 years. The main studies were undertaken from the period of the early 1970's to the early 1980's (Altschul 1972; Cormack 1976, 1983; Towell 1975; Carr 1979). In addition, a number of studies on a smaller scale, which are of relevance in this section, have been documented (Macilwaine 1983; Bunch 1985; Brooking 1986). Butterworth (1991) points out that only Macilwaine's (1983) and Carr's (1979) studies have sought to describe the work of mental health nurses in psychiatric units of general hospitals.

The recently published review of mental health nursing (DOH 1994), the first major review since the report "Psychiatric Nursing: Today and Tomorrow" in 1968 (Ministry of Health 1968), has added to this existing body of knowledge.

Various aspects of the work of mental health nurses have been looked at, either exploring in general their role and skills, or looking at particular aspects, such as the therapeutic relationship, or elements of that relationship, for example empathy.

Early studies examined how nurses distributed their time among various general categories of activity (Oppenheim 1955; John 1961). These studies revealed little of the underlying understanding and meaning that guides nurses in their work. Macilwaine (1983) questions the validity of these "work-study" types of research, arguing that the categories systems used seemed to be the work of people entirely unfamiliar with the role of the mental health nurse. She adds that the lack of any theoretical perspective or guiding principle makes any data difficult to interpret, as there is no definition of nurse behaviours likely to be of benefit to the patient.

Altschul's (1972) study has generally been recognised as revolutionary and of considerable importance (Towell 1975; Macilwaine 1983). Her work could be described as the first major piece of research exploring the dyadic interaction patterns between nurse and patient. She wondered whether it was possible to find any connection between the frequency and duration of the interactions, and the formation of a relationship. She found that factors such as the patient's age, gender, diagnosis and behaviour, and the nurse's gender and professional qualifications all played a role in determining the frequency and duration of the interactions. She could however not find any evidence of a prevailing treatment ideology among nurses, nor any theoretical basis upon which nurses acted in their dyadic interactions.

Altschul (1972), whose study was influenced by Peplau's (1952) interpersonal relations constructs, could be criticised for assuming that nurses in this country would have developed the qualities and skills she was looking for. Indeed, it has been pointed out that British nurses were rarely taught specific theoretical approaches to patients (Macilwaine 1983). Altschul (1972) herself admitted that her focus on dyadic interactions may have been alien to the nurses' habitual mode of thinking.

Towell (1975) adopting an illuminative approach to the study of mental health nursing, concluded that the occupational label 'psychiatric nurse' encompassed a cluster of roles, depending on the setting in which these were performed. On admission wards, he observed that nurses played a key linking role between patients and most aspects of hospital arrangements in a ward organised for medical servicing. As far as personal relationships were concerned, nurses lacked both the support and the theorectical perspective which would have been required to make use of such relationaships as an explicit contribution to patient treatment. He appeared to confirm Altschul's (1972) earlier findings of the limited extent of the role of personal relationships with patients.

Towell (1975), commenting on the increased concentration of psychiatric facilities in general hospital locations, also observed that the culture of the general hospital may impose restraints on the approaches realised. Indeed, he found that nurse interactions were influenced by the treatment ideology, for example nurses interpreted patient behaviours on the basis of medical diagnostic categories.

Cormack (1976) assumed in his study that if nurses performed a psychotherapeutic or counselling role, then this performance would involve verbal communication with patients, and that this performance could be measured and described. Through observation he found that nurses spent 13% of their time in verbal communication, but that the content was mainly social, and concerned with the patient's psychiatric state, treatment and progress. In his examination of the nurse-patient relationship, he could find no evidence that the nurse was personally and actively attempting to function as a treatment form.

Cormack (1976) could be criticised for failing to observe nurse-patient interactions within a clear psychotherapeutic framework. The quantitative nature of his study prevented Cormack from exploring the context in which these interactions took place. He explained his findings by making reference to the discrepancies between the prescribed literature and nurse training, which, as he himself indicated, included very little teaching in the way of counselling and psychotherapeutic skills. As a counter argument he put forward the idea that nurses may have made a deliberate choice not to follow the prescribed role. However, it appears that yet again a study was conducted on misconceived assumptions, in this case however these were known, but apparently ignored, before the study began.

In addition to the educational explanation, Cormack (1976) also proposed organisational and ideological explanations, pointing out that nurses' administrative duties frequently disrupted one to one interactions. This prevented them from having prolonged contact with patients. Drawing on the work of Strauss et al (1964) he found that nurses adopted whichever ideology was professed by the medical staff.

Although Cormack (1976) did not find evidence of a deliberate planned approach to their therapeutic work, he hypothesised that what mental health nurses do could be seen as a valuable form of unsystematic and unrecognised therapy, which presumably is waiting to be unravelled to identify what the essential ingredients are of a caring therapeutic relationship.

Carr (1979) some years later found the interaction in the nurse-patient situation equally ill-defined. On the basis of his study, which described the role of mental health nurses on an acute admission unit of a general hospital, he suggested that the suitability of these units as places for caring for acutely disturbed people needed to be assessed, expressing surprise that little or no work appeared to have been carried out in this area.

In a second study Cormack (1983) attempted to describe effective actions and behaviours of ward based mental health nurses through the collection and analysis of critical incidents. He found that differences in shift, speciality and grade had a minimal influence on their actions and behaviours. However, he highlighted a number of methodological shortcomings. He pointed out that what people write and what they do may be two different things. He also suggested that nurses may have found it difficult to describe specific elements of their role. Finally, he questioned whether it is possible to identify what effective and ineffective nursing behaviours are, as there are no criteria available by which to measure these.

Macilwaine (1983) concentrated her study on the relationship between the mental health nurse and the neurotic patient. Her study was set in the acute admission unit of a general hospital. Of the 200 tape recorded incidents collected, 36% were identified as administrative interactions. However, she failed to acknowledge that the independent judges were unable to categorise 40% of the interactions. Ignoring this discrepancy, Macilwaine (1983) claimed that care was given on an ad hoc basis, and that talking to patients tended to have a low priority. She argued that giving patients a series of brief interactions to provide them with emotional support was no substitute for a planned programme of therapeutic interventions. She concluded that if mental health nurses are to act as therapeutic agents, they should have specific skills and positive attitudes to deal with a range of psychiatric problems. She had found no evidence of these characteristics in her study. It is interesting to note Rolfe's (1990) recent small scale study, in which he found little evidence of therapeutic attitudes among RMN students.

Bunch (1985) explored and described the way that hospital based mental health nurses are affected by the abnormal communication used by schizophrenic patients. Her study was set in a framework of structural requirements that influenced nurses' work. These structural requirements contained three elements: a professional, clinical, and institutional requirement, which respectively referred to the ideology and goals of mental health nursing, the expectations about skills and abilities, and the expectations, norms and rules of the organisation.

Bunch (1985) found that nurses focused on institutional business when talking to patients. The institutional requirements appeared to override both the professional and clinical requirements, suggesting that bureaucracy stifles the endeavours of nurses to communicate therapeutically. Lutzen (1990) arrived at similar conclusions, pointing out that personal values and ideologies conflicted sharply with the values and ideologies of the institution.

Emrich (1989) employed a transactional analysis framework in her exploration of the nurse-patient relationship. Her findings showed that nurses tended to use a parental interactional style, contradicting the notion that these interactions are confirming and open. It is interesting to note that interactions between patients showed more evidence of health promoting responses. In addition to the explanations offered by earlier authors, Emrich (1989) suggested that the fast pace of an acute setting may lead nurses to deal with patients in what they perceive to be the most efficient manner.

The ability to show or express empathy is considered to be one of the essential attributes of the mental health nurse in the establishment of a therapeutic relationship. Gallop et al (1990) examined the empathic skills of 113 mental health nurses through a staff-patient interaction scale, which consisted of a list of statements requiring a response. They identified three categories of responses, with 20% offering no care, 51% offering solutions, and 29% expressing affective involvement. On the basis of these findings they claim that nurse provided quick solutions to immediate problems, such as giving advice or making supportive statements, rather than aiming to understand the patient's subjective experience. It could be argued that the respondents were not offered a context, thereby rendering their responses meaningless. In addition, the use of such scales did not inform about actual behaviour. The authors however concluded that there was little evidence that nurses were committed to the values of empathic skills, and wondered whether remedicalization of mental health care may have lead them to abandon the exploration of feelings.

The assumption that nurses possessed or were taught these skills was used by Cox (1990) to criticise Gallop's et al (1990) work. She claimed that nurses were not rewarded for displaying empathy, arguing that the message was being conveyed by other disciplines that valuable work was only accomplished within the context of structured

20

psychotherapeutic sessions, thereby reinforcing the lower value that nurses may have attached to their empathetic skills.

Finally, a recent study by Handy (1991) appeared to bring together and confirm the majority of the findings identified by the previous authors. An analysis of the activities of mental health nurses showed that 33% of their time was spent on paperwork and continuous telephone conversations, which, she suggested, gave nurses a legitimate excuse for avoiding patient contact. Although half of their time was spent in direct patient contact, this related to mainly practical tasks, such as the administration of medication and the supervision of meals. She observed that the seniority of nursing staff inversely related to the amount of time spend with patients, with the charge nurse spending 15% of her/his time in direct patient contact, and nursing assistants spending 60% of their time with patients. She highlighted a general tendency for patients to be dealt with by least qualified staff with less knowledge of these patients. She further found that interactions were initiated on an ad hoc basis, with nurses tending to terminate these conversations after relatively brief periods, only to retire to the security of the nursing office. Analysis of nurses' diaries however led Handy (1991) to conclude that effective therapeutic relationships were attempted, but stifled, doomed to failure within the medically oriented environment.

It seems that this review of the literature has highlighted a number of recurrent themes, that appear to influence the development of an identity for hospital based mental health nurses as prescribed and promoted in the literature and in educational establishments. It may also have shed some light on the reasons behind the confusion about the position of mental health nurses in that setting.

Almost all the studies reviewed seem to have started from the premise, rightly or wrongly, that therapeutic relationships and interactions are beneficial and valuable for patients, and that mental health nurses possess a range of skills that can positively influence the mental health status of those patients.

The findings in those studies appear to indicate a number of factors that influence, mainly negatively, how nurses practise mental health nursing. Ideological differences, interprofessional and intraprofessional conflicts, administrative duties, educational deficiencies, bureaucratic constraints, organisational structures, personal inabilities and unwillingness, low status, environmental unsuitability, and managerial pressures have all been identified to explain why some nurses do not perform as prescribed and promoted in the literature. Keltner (1985) points out that nursing experts often claim that the incongruence between the "real" and the "ideal" is the practising nurse's problem. This review seems to suggest that this claim is too simplistic, and only part of the story.

What still does not seem clear is what nurses themselves think about their roles, their skills, and position in acute mental health care.

3 The methodology

In this chapter the methodology of the study will be presented, which will incorporate an outline of the sampling method, access to the participants, and the methods of data collection and analysis used.

This is a descriptive study, which has a qualitative nature through its methods of data collection and analysis. These methods are respectively the semi-structured interview and thematic content analysis. It has been argued that strictly speaking there is no such thing as qualitative research, there are only qualitative data (Tesch 1990).

Descriptive studies are marked by minimal interpretation and conceptualisation, written in such a way as to allow readers to draw their own conclusions and generalisations (Taylor and Bogdan 1984). It would be misleading to suggest that these studies write themselves. The researcher presents and orders the data according to what he thinks is important. Emerson (1983) refers to descriptions that present in close detail the context and meanings of events that are relevant to those involved in them.

The sample

The sample in this study was drawn from qualified registered mental health nurses, working in an acute psychiatric admission unit of a district hospital, and from other health professionals employed in that setting:

psychologists, social workers, occupational therapists and psychiatrists. This group will be referred to as the non-nurse respondents. Including these other disciplines was a response to Cormack's (1983) suggestion of incorporating their perceptions when exploring the skills of mental health nurses.

The nature and methodology of the study warranted the adoption of a non-probability sample. Due to the constraints of time a pre-determined sample of 16 respondents was decided upon, made up of 8 nurses and 8 non-nurse respondents. Morse's (1991) suggestion was borne in mind. She pointed out that the sample needs to be both appropriate and adequate, i.e. the choice should "fit" the purpose and be able to generate sufficient quality data. A purposive sample was used, in which individuals thought to be most important or relevant to the topic under investigation, were targeted for the research (Sommer and Sommer 1991). Within this framework, a volunteer sample procedure was adopted, in which people willing to participate were approached, or were given the opportunity to approach the researcher. A shortcoming of this approach is its self selected nature, with only those willing to participate giving perhaps a distorted view of the topic under examination. Sandelowski (1986) in this context refers to "elite bias". However, it has been suggested that it is exactly the purpose and intent to find respondents with knowledge of the subject (Morse 1991).

The sample of nurse volunteers was then stratified by clinical grading, to ensure an even distribution across the grades. This process was not relevant for the sample of the non-nurse respondents.

The sample then came from a local, easy accessible pool of people, with a willingness to participate. The sample was known, to varying degrees, to the researcher in his capacity as nurse tutor. This prior knowledge may have influenced the process and outcome of the study, an issue which will be addressed later in this chapter.

Selecting the sample

Contact with the potential pool of nurses was established via the Director of Nursing Services (DNS) and the Senior Nurse Manager (Acute) of the Mental Health Unit. Access was granted to contact the ward managers of the two admission ward to set up the study. A list of the nursing establishment, by grade, was given to the researcher to help identify possible candidates. Communications proved to be poor. Ward staff had not been informed of my intentions as promised by the Senior Nurse Manager, which delayed the selection process. Eventually however, ward managers were briefed and potential candidates identified. Some were excluded due to being on permanent night shift, sick leave or annual leave. Interested candidates were invited to contact the researcher rather than the other way round, to avoid undue pressure and influence to participate. This again delayed the process, but was considered unavoidable. A sample of 8 nurses, with various lengths of experience, and made up of different grades and gender, was eventually selected. All expressed a keen interest, although some may have volunteered because of the opportunity to offload their frustration and anger. As one respondent pointed out: "it's about time some work was done in this area."

Access to the potential pool of the other disciplines took various forms. Initially, Heads of the respective Departments were contacted by telephone. The occupational therapists and social workers expressed an immediate interest and volunteers were quickly identified. The District psychologist was on annual leave, and the researcher was invited to write stating his intentions. It took several reminders, but a month later, a number of psychologists had volunteered.

The most difficult discipline to establish contact with proved to be the psychiatrists. Their secretaries, acting as gate-keepers, responded to the numerous phone calls with a consistent:

I've passed your message on, and they'll be in touch soon.
The secretary of one of the psychiatrists eventually informed the researcher that he (the psychiatrist) was too busy to participate. Another psychiatrist was met by chance on one of the wards. Reminding him of the request, he too responded that he was too busy. Psychiatrists from a neighbouring admission unit were then approached, who had no hesitation in participating in the research.

A sample of 8 health professionals, drawn from the four disciplines, was thus established.

Method of data collection

It has been argued that no method is equally suited for all purposes (Taylor and Bogdan 1984). Research methods are determined by research interests and aims, the circumstances of the setting or the people to be studied, and the practical constraints faced by the researcher. This led to the choice of the semi-structured, audio-taped interview.

Brenner et al (1985) point out that the interview is one of the most widely used methods in social research. The type of interview adopted for this study has been described as semi-structured (Sommer and Sommer 1991), in-depth (Taylor and Bogdan 1984), exploratory (Oppenheim 1992) and account interviewing (Brenner 1985). This qualitative method of interviewing has been defined as:

> "a face to face encounter between researcher and informant, directed towards understanding the informant's perspectives on their lives, experiences or situations as expressed in their own words." (Taylor and Bogdan 1984:77).

Within this semi-structured approach, in which the interviewer becomes the research instrument, there is a clear frame of reference in which the respondents are asked similar questions (see Appendix 1). The order and manner in which these questions are asked and answered may differ from person to person. Indeed, it has been noted that although the research purposes are governed by the questions asked, the respondents control the content, sequence and wording (Cohen and Manion 1985).

Advantages of this method

Allport's (1942) dictum that if you wanted to know something about people's activities, the best way of finding out was to ask them, remains as relevant today.

The central value of this approach is that it allows both the interviewer and respondent to explore and clarify the meaning of the questions and answers, thereby providing opportunities to pursue half answered questions and encourage more detailed responses. Within a framework, determined by the interviewer, sufficient openness and flexibility are allowed to help to illuminate the thoughts, feelings and experiences of the respondent around the topic under investigation. This flexible nature may in turn increase rapport and facilitate a smooth interaction, thereby enhancing the chance of obtaining in-depth information.

Limitations of this method

There is now a growing awareness of the limitations of the interview as a method of data collection. Brenner et al (1985) refer to areas such as distortions in data transformation, opportunities for bias, and lack of conceptual schemes to aid interpretation. It could be argued that these last two limitations equally apply to the method of data analysis.

The most quoted limitation seems to be that what people say they do is not always the same as what people do, as has been suggested, people say and do things in different situations (Taylor and Bogdan 1984).

Walker (1983) observes that people may also find it hard to break out of the constraints of telling you what they think you want, or ought, to know, in order to tell you what you want to hear.

The information obtained through interview is limited to the spoken word. It may be that people are not always able to express their thoughts and ideas, as Polanyi (1967) has observed. Brenner (1985) adds that respondents have to select from their past experiences those aspects that seem significant and worth reporting. In other words, what do respondents consider to be relevant, and what can the respondent remember? Others have pointed out that respondents may be reluctant to articulate their thoughts (Taylor and Bogdan 1984).

Distortions may also be influenced by the interviewer. As the interviewer becomes the research instrument, an awareness of preconceived ideas, but also an awareness of his own interpersonal skills and qualities is important. Finally, a number of other factors have been identified that will inhibit or enhance the process and outcome of the interview. Oppenheim (1992) refers to the gender, age, background and culture of both the interviewer and respondent, while others have pointed out mood, desire to please, and ulterior motives (Footwhyte 1982), appearance and acceptance (Measor 1985) and the wider context of the interview (Burgess 1984).

It was with these various factors and influences in mind that the interviews were conducted.

The interview process

Prior to the start of each interview, respondents were informed about the length of the interview (between 30-45 minutes). They were given, in addition to the explanation provided on first contact, a verbal outline of the topic area and method of analysis. With hindsight, it may have been more beneficial to have provided the respondents in advance with a written outline of the context, as many respondents reflected aloud with "I haven't really thought about that" to some of the questions posed. More in-depth information may have been collected in that way. However, this lack of prior context enhanced the spontaneity and gave a useful insight into the manner they constructed their world and the situation in which they found themselves.

Each respondent was asked, at initial contact, and again at the start of the interview, permission to have the interview recorded on audiotape. They were informed that only the respondent, the interviewer, his supervisor and an independent judge would have access to this tape. All but two of the respondents agreed to this arrangement. In these two cases brief notes were taken during the interview, which were transcribed immediately after the interview. The audiotapes were transcribe in full. These were a literal representation of the words spoken during the interview, in the order that they were spoken (Burnard and Morrison 1990). Pauses, intonations and emphases were excluded, although observations and perceptions about the respondent were noted immediately after each interview. The transcripts were returned to the respondents as soon as possible for verification. It also offered them a further opportunity to add to, delete or change the contents of their spoken text.

It was thought essential to audiotape the interviews. Oppenheim (1992) points out that the contents can be examined by more than one person, and examined more than once, thereby increasing the validity of later analysis. Having the full transcript available also reduced the possible bias and distortion through the interviewer's interpretation of the text. In addition, it allowed for a better concentration on the process of the interview, rather than trying to remember what respondents were saying.

However, it has been suggested that the interviewer may cease to listen carefully (Brenner 1985). Sommer and Sommer (1991) do not recommend their use either, arguing that it is intrusive, may make respondents uncomfortable, and may compromise confidentiality. Indeed, there was some initial embarrassment, with one respondent commenting "do I have to listen to it?", but on the whole respondents seemed at ease.

A further drawback of using an audiotape was the time it took to transcribe. Each 30-45 minute interview took approximately three hours to transcribe. Each tape was labelled, coded by number, date and length of interview. Additional notes were made immediately after each interview of observations that had not been captured by the audiotape.

Walker (1983) comments that the kind of questions asked are often enough to set off thoughts into the respondent's head, that do not stop when the interview ends. Indeed, some respondents commented, on returning the transcript to the researcher, that "the interview had been very thought provoking and had raised lots of questions", thanking the researcher for the opportunity to have been able to participate.

At the end of the interview, each respondent was invited to add anything that may have been of relevance to the study. Some did, making useful connections, expanding on earlier comments, or introducing new ones.

The interviews were conducted over a period of three months. Finding a mutually convenient time accounted for most of this length of time. All the interviews took place within the respondent's work environment, either in their office or, in the case of most of the nurses, in a quiet room on the ward. On three occasions the interviews were interrupted by the telephone.

The existing nurse tutor-practitioner relationship influenced the newly established interviewer-interviewee relationship. This was illustrated by one nurse, who informed me shortly before the start of the interview that he had "read up" the night before, in case he did not know the answers to my questions! It may be that he perceived it as a "test". Others seemed to have come with their own agendas and did not appear to respond to some of the questions, but made sure I heard what they thought I needed to know, not in my capacity as a researcher, but in my role as nurse tutor.

Method of data analysis

There are many styles of analysis that are called content analysis. The method used to analyse the interview data in this study is based on and adapted from a variety of approaches (Glaser and Strauss 1967; Taylor and Bogdan 1984; Mostyn 1985; Berg 1989; Riley 1990; Crabtree and Miller 1992) and has been described as thematic content analysis (Burnard 1991).

The aim of this approach was to look for meaningful relationships in the data and to arrive at a detailed and systematic identification of themes and linking these under a reasonably exhaustive category system. To strengthen the validity of these categories, the transcripts were ready by two independent judges, who arrived at broadly similar categories as the researcher.

No attempt was made to analyse the data from a particular theoretical standpoint, for example psycho-analytical perspective. The intention was to describe, interpret and give meaning to the overt content, and to try to understand the skills, roles and position of nurses in an acute psychiatric environment, as perceived by the respondents.

Initial analysis, searching for themes and patterns, took place after each interview. These were incorporated in subsequent interviews, in order to confirm or disconfirm these early ideas. There was then a phase of simultaneous collection and analysis of the data. However, the main analysis process took place once all the data had been collected.

Two copies of each hand-written transcript were used to work with the data, while the original was filed. All the transcripts, 150 pages of text with a 2" left margin, were read to gain a sense of the data and identify possible themes and categories. Notes were made in the margin (see Appendix 2). This process of open coding was repeated twice. At this stage the two independent judges confirmed their categories.

Subsequent coding was achieved by reading the text again, using a number of coloured highlighting pens to refine the coding of the categories. These sections were identified in the margin by page and interview number, in order to trace the original source. These coded elements of text, which contained sentences and phrases, to stay close to the original intentions of the respondent, were then cut and pasted. The second copy was left intact to maintain the context of the coded sections. It was at this stage important to "make the codes fit the data, rather than the data fit the codes" (Taylor and Bogdan 1984:136).

The reorganised data was then read again and further sub-categories identified, using the same process as described above. The final process of writing up then took place, with the original transcripts and audiotapes at hand to stay close to the intentions of the respondents.

Taylor and Bogdan (1984) suggest that the researcher should give the readers enough information how the research was conducted to enable them to discount the findings. Using this process of content analysis, as indeed with all forms of analysis, the researcher needed to be aware of a number of issues that may have influenced the reliability and validity of the data. Reordering raw material into reliable and valid data is open to researcher bias. Describing the method used may, in some way, address Cicourel's (1964) concern, who argues that although content analysis implies the expectation that meaningful patterns may exist in communication, its significance cannot be assumed only by virtue of its categorisation. How the researcher decides what his categories are, and how they are to be used by reference to the theoretical presuppositions inherent in the method of analysis needs to be made explicit.

The themes and categories that emerged were partly deter-mined by the questions asked, partly arrived at through the researcher's knowledge and understanding of the topic under investigation, and partly through validation by independent judges. Miles and Huber-man's (1984) concern for "holistic fallacy", making the data look more congruent and patterned than they are, served as a constant reminder to work with the data as given. An open mind was kept to the data, although it was difficult to shed the "baggage" that the researcher inevitably carried with him.

Coding, analysing and writing up the results may seem a straightforward process, but the decision of what to include and what to exclude, and at the same time remaining as close and as truthful to the intentions of the respondents, was a difficult process. Decisions had to be made what could be classified as "dross" (Field and Morse 1985). Meanings that people attach to the words they use had at times to be assumed (Burnard 1991). Assumptions that the most frequent patterns discovered in the text are also the most relevant had to be made. This suggests that it is always difficult to find a reliable and

valid method. Ultimately, the responsibility rests with the researcher to provide an honest and clear account of the meaning of the words expressed by the respondents, and one which provides a fair representation of their world. External validity, or "fittingness" as Guba and Lincoln (1981) prefer to call it, may be achieved if this representation is recognised by prospective readers as meaningful and applicable in terms of their own experiences.

Alternatives and objections to the content analysis approach

The preceding sections of this chapter have described how the data in this study were collected and analysed. In this section, we explore other ways of thinking about data in qualitative analysis. Further to the discussions offered here, an example of the beginnings of a reanalysis of one of the interviews is offered as an appendix.

Nurse researchers frequently use qualitative research methods (see, for example, Oiler 1982, Munhall and Oiler 1986, Abrahams 1984, Field and Morse 1986, Chenitz and Swanson 1986). The aim of qualitative researcher, it has been claimed, is to describe the *sorts* of experiences and events that there may be in the world (Cormack, 1984, Bryman 1988). Qualitative research is usually characterized as involving 'soft' findings, as rejecting the positivist paradigm (however that might be defined) and offering an attempt at representing the 'lived experience' of respondents - the everyday, 'ordinary' and subjective experience of the person who is, at all times, immersed in his or her own world (Ashworth, Giorgi, and de Koning, 1986, van Manen 1977). Data are usually in the form of text and most often this text is in the form of interview transcripts (although other sorts of data presentation are available(Berg 1989, Fink and Kosekoff 1985)). This section, however, concentrates, specifically on textual data and textual data, for the purposes of this section is any data that takes the form of sentences and paragraphs of information in a written or printed format.

Once the qualitative researcher has collected data, he or she has, of necessity, to make sense of those data. Perhaps the only 'pure' way (and this purity may also be called into question) might be to present a set of interview transcripts as they stand. In this way, respondents, it might be argued, are represented most accurately and 'in their own words'. All that would have to happen would be that the reader would be invited to 'make sense' of the transcripts. It should be noted, at this point, at what is being suggested here: the reader might be called upon to *interpret* the unadulterated data in any way that he or she may choose - there would be no 'signposts' offered by the researcher. However, most researchers would be unwilling to take such an approach. The argument would probably be put forward that binding up interview transcripts in this way would not constitute 'doing research'. It would be further argued that 'research' necessarily involves some analysis of data and some interpretation of it. In all forms of qualitative method that the current writers could find, qualitative analysis *always* involves some *reduction* of the text. If the whole of the text cannot stand on its own, then it follows that some (or much) reduction *must* take place. It follows, too, that, if this happens, the researcher must make decisions about what is included for analysis and what is left out. Indeed, Field and More (1986), fairly uncritically, use the term 'dross' to describe those elements of data that are not 'important' to the research. The finding of 'dross' seems unlikely to be a scientific enterprise but one that exercises the researcher's personal judgment. Also, it may be argued that 'meanings' are not only found in the more 'important' statements that people make but also in the 'fillers', the repetitions and the idiosyncrasies of everyday speech. Also, in passing, it can be noted that the notion of 'dross' is a derogatory one and it use suggests that the researcher is already adopting a particular value judgement vis a vis the interview transcripts.

A caveat may be added, at this stage, that the term 'reductionism' may have, at least, two meanings. First, it can be used to denote a process in which phenomena are broken down into constituent parts. Second, it can be used to suggest a process by which phenomena are 'reduced' and distilled in order to attempt to get at their 'essences'. It is the second sort that is being discussed here.

Analysis of textual data

There have been various methods devised for analyzing textual data (see, for example, Miles and Huberman 1994, Field and Morse 1986, Bell and Newby 1977, Berg 1989). There is the grounded theory approach in which it is argued that 'categories' can be allowed to 'emerge' out of the textual data and that once such categories have been identified, pieces of text from a range of documents can be brought together under category headings (Glaser and Strauss 1967, Strauss 1987). Other methods invite the research to 'immerse' him or herself in the data in order to identify hidden (or overt) meanings of the text (Ashworth, Giorgi and de Koning 1986). In this form of data analysis, the belief seems to be that if the research can soak up enough of the text he or she will find its 'essence'. Smith (1992) makes the interesting observation that the terms *ethnography, field methods, qualitative inquiry, participant observation, case study, naturalistic methods,* and *responsive evaluation* have become practically synonymous, suggesting a great similarity between a whole range of apparently different qualitative methods of data collection. If this is the case, then it follows that *data analysis* methods are likely to be similar.

Sometimes, too, there is a search for the *validity* of the analysis - although this is an area that is notoriously contentious (Kirk and Miller 1986). Some writers recommend that the researcher invites other researchers or even the respondents to explore the data and, in this way, to 'validate' (or otherwise) the researchers category systems (Field and Morse 1986). Other methods include the more quantitative one of content analysis in which words and phrases are identified and counted (Krippendorf 1980). Sometimes, it is recommended that a range of methods be used (Silverman 1986).

This is by no means an exhaustive listing of the types of textual data analysis methods that are currently recommended but to point to some of the characteristics that define qualitative analytical methods.

Whatever method of analysis is used, it will usually be found that most or all of the following characteristics are present:

- the researcher reduces the volume of the text
- the researcher searches for categories or types of responses
- the researcher groups together 'similar' types of utterances or ideas
- the 'similar' utterances or ideas are brought together in a report of the findings
- attempts (sometimes elaborate attempts) are made to 'stay true' to the text and to the imputed meanings offered by the respondent.

The overall aim of qualitative analysis appears to be the finding of coherent patterns of ideas, thoughts, utterances, beliefs and so on. Perhaps the most extreme form of 'pattern finding' in the qualitative research literature can be found in Miles and Huberman (1994) who describe various ways of 'arranging' patterns of data by using various methods of analysis and by compiling various 'maps' of the data.

Some writers insist of attempting to find ways of 'purifying' the method of finding these discrete elements. One such example of an attempt is that of 'bracketing' (in a certain type of phenomenological research) (Kvale 1983). Here, the researcher is asked to set aside his or her own beliefs, feelings, values and so forth in order to see more clearly and more objectively the beliefs, ideas and so on that are in the data. In many senses, then, the qualitative researcher is trying to replicate many of the working methods of the quantitative researcher. The qualitative researcher who attempts to adopt a 'clean' approach to the data might be seen as trying not to 'contaminate' the findings. He or she is attempting to adopt an objective position vis a vis the data. It is suggested, here, that all of these sorts of attempts are mistaken in their approach - and for the following reasons.

First and arguably, there are no 'hidden' or 'real' meanings embedded in text. Text is made up of groups of words and we can never be sure that the words that are found in (for example) interview transcripts do or do not capture the 'real meanings' of the respondent. The respondent might easily have chosen 'other' words and the way that he or she is *using* words may not respond to the researcher's view of what the words mean. Nor does checking back with the respondent cover this criticism, for once the researcher raises the possibility of a particular category system with the respondent, that researcher is 'leading' the respondent in a particular direction. Now this may not matter - but it does show how 'slippery' words and meanings are. If the respondent *can* be lead in this way, it suggests that the *written* words that are captured in the original text are not, necessarily, a profound expression of that respondent's true beliefs but merely a set of words offered at a particular meaning in time. They may or may not 'mean' anything. But to work away at those words as if to distill them into 'essence' or particular 'meanings' may be to overload the text and to embark on a search for 'truth' that is spurious. Also, meanings are never contained only in the words that are used but in the patterns of words, the emphases, the pauses, the facial expressions of the speaker and so on. Leys (1986) sums up some of the problems of what constitutes 'communication' as follows:

> Not only can the message reach its destination without having to be fully spelled out, but it is precisely because it is not fully spelled out that it can reach its destination. (Leys 1986 p29).

If we try to hard at analyzing what people 'really mean', we are likely to find that meaning elusive, just as it can be noted that if we attempt to understand every word of a dialogue taking place in a film or play, we are likely to loose the thread of what is being said. Close attention to text will not, of itself, yield up more accurate meanings of that text. Virginia Woolf described the difficult of the fact that words can yield so many different meanings and associations:

> Take the simple sentence 'Passing Russell Square'. That proved useless because besides the surface meaning it contained so many sunken meanings. The word 'passing' suggested the transciency of things, the passing of time and the changes of human life. Then the word 'Russell' suggested the rustling of leaves and the skirt on a polished floor; also the ducal house of Bedford and half the history of England. Finally the word 'Square' brings in the sight, the shape of an actual square combined with some visual suggestions of the stark angularity of stucco. Thus one sentence of the simplest kind rouses the imagination, the memory, the eye and the ear - all combine in reading it. (Woolf 1961 p 173).

Also, understanding of meaning also involves an appreciation of metaphor, irony, humour and of the speaker's belief systems and of the way in which he or she uses words. And all of these points can be misunderstood - and, arguably, very *easily* misunderstood by the researcher. No amount of pondering on the written word can guarantee that the researcher can access the intended meaning of the respondent. Nor, of course, can it be guaranteed that any given interview will contain what the respondent 'really means'. He or she may, for example, be unable to express him or herself clearly, he or she may exaggerate or lie, he may be 'lead' by the researcher, he or she may be affected by what he or she things the researcher wants to hear and so on. Lyotard identifies some of the problems of understanding text 'after the event' as follows:

> Hence the fact that work and text have the characters of an *event*; hence they always come too late for their author, or, what amounts to the same thing, their being put into work, their realization...always begins too soon (Lyotard 1983 p 73).

The texts that are the written transcriptions of interview tapes are no longer, necessarily, accurate representations of those interviews. The fact that others are reading the transcripts means that those 'others' bring their own meanings to the text. The interviewee, as it were, no longer 'owns' the text. In this sense, then, the reader 'writes' the text and that text is 'reinvented' each time it is read by a different reader and, quite possibly, reinvented by the same reader, returning to the text. Certainly, the interviewee no longer has any control over how the text may or may not be interpreted.

And yet many qualitative researchers depend - as their only source of data - on 'one off', fairly short, interviews. After this, they compound the problem, by squeezing the data for hidden meaning and then drawing conclusions from this process.

Another approach may be simply to acknowledge that any given interview that is transcribed leads to the production of *text* - words - both interesting and varied on the page. However, the *veracity* of those words is always in dispute. And this is a vital issue. If the truth value of the words on the page is in dispute, then any *analysis* of the words is also in dispute. The qualitative research could find him or herself compounding error upon error - and all this in a search for what is 'really going on'. If the 'truth content' of a transcript is 'slippery', then any attempt at analyzing it is bound to lead to further 'slipperiness'. Miles, sums up, in a more general, way, the problems that are faced all the way through the analysis processes in qualitative studies:

> The most serious and central difficult in the use of qualitative data is that methods of analysis are not well formulated. For

quantitative data, there are clear conventions the research can use. But the analyst faced with a bank of qualitative data has very few guidelines for protection against self-delusion, let alone the presentation of unreliable or invalid conclusions to scientific or policy-making audiences. How can we be sure that an 'earthy', 'undeniable', 'serendipitous' finding is not, in fact, *wrong*? (Miles 1979, p 581).

A change of emphasis

At this point, it becomes important to change the emphasis. It is suggested here that an alternative (and valid) way of viewing texts is *not* to concentrate on what the respondent may or may not have 'meant' (for the moment in which we might have discerned what was meant has passed, both for the researcher and for the respondent). As Lyotard, above, has suggested, the text arrives 'too late'. Instead, the researcher may concentrate on what meanings *the researcher* brings to the text. In a sense, this has always happened. It is impossible to read text without, also, 'interpreting it'. A 'low level' of interpretation might be of the variety in which the researcher acknowledges 'I understand the words that this person is using'. A 'high level' of interpretation might be where the researcher views the words through a particular theoretical framework. For example, the psychodynamic researcher might 'see' the data from a psychodynamic point of view and the 'interpretation', at this level, would be of the variety in which intentions and meanings were imputed. Thus, there may be a dimension of interpretation, ranging from the concrete to the highly abstract. Along that dimension, many shades of interpretation are impossible.

This is an important shift of emphasis. The point, being, that there is never *one* interpretation that may be made of a text but always *many*. Further, there is, it may be argued, no *right* interpretation nor even 'more accurate' interpretation - only *different* interpretation and at different degrees of abstraction. All of this is based on the idea that a) it is impossible to understand the 'insides of peoples' minds' through their utterances, b) it is impossible to impute peoples' intentions and meanings directly from written transcripts of their interviews and c) people's beliefs, ideas, feelings and so on are in a constant state of flux. To represent *this* set of interviews as being in some way

38

representative of 'what this group of people really mean' is fallacious. A moment's reflection will reveal that all people are shifting and inconsistent in 'what they really mean'. Neither one nor many interviews will get the researcher nearer to what a person really means and the quest for such 'real meaning' is erroneous. What any human being 'means' changes according to a huge range of variables, including, at least, their mood, their current situation, their life style, what they have just been thinking about, looking at, talking to, doing and so on. All of these variables will be further affected by the presence (or otherwise) of the interviewer.

Transcripts as stories

Given these variables, instead of viewing interview transcripts as records of the sorts of things that people *mean*, it might be useful to view interview transcripts as narratives or stories. They are stories that the respondent puts together during the dynamic of the interview. In other interviews, with other researchers, the story might be a different one. On a different day, in a different situation, the story might be different again. None of this matters if it is accepted that *exploring* those stories might give us insight into some parts of the human condition, in much the same way as novels and other forms of fiction can capture parts of the human condition. What brings both of these forms together is that they are both 'written' by human beings and they both draw upon and reflect human experience.

How, then, might such a researcher proceed? First, he or she would have to abandon notions of objectivity, of a particular method and of attempting to find 'essences'. Instead, he or she might explore the whole of each transcript and to find *as many explanations for the text as possible*. In this form of analysis, the researcher might explore the meanings of words, the concepts that were described, the metaphors that were used, the pictures that were evoked and so on. The interpretation would thus be 'thick' and never subject to validity checks for their might be huge numbers of possible interpretations and it would never be the intention to focus on the respondent's 'hidden meanings'. The 'meanings', if there are any, would be the *researcher's* rather than the respondents.

A recapitulation may help at this point. It has been argued that there is no reason why a textual document may contain particular meanings and that it may be important to acknowledge this and for the researcher to concentrate on the meanings that the *researcher* brings to the text. All meanings, by virtue of their being no way of arbitrating, may be valid. In this formulation, there is no consensus to be reached and it may, or course, be the case that the reader of the final research report might bring yet another set of meanings to bear on the work that he or she reads. Again, this second level reading may inform the reader just as the reading of the transcripts informed the researcher. Gradually, and in a seemingly arbitrary way, there would be a building up of a rich and varied 'evidence' about the human condition. It would be the opposite of reductionism and the encouragement of pluralism. At its worst, it might be viewed as 'research anarchy' and, at its best, it may be seen as a fresh way of thinking about the things people talk about. For, in an important sense, what has been described above echoes what many people do in a conversation.

If two people are discussing a topic, one may assert something. The other may then refute it, think about it, agree with it, dissect it or otherwise analyze it - and respond. This response is then 'digested' by the first person, who adds another 'layer of meaning' to what has been said. In this way, the dialogue - and the ideas - develop. There are no 'real meanings' hidden in the dialogue. No one, usually, attempts to thrash out what the other person 'really means'. Each, instead, makes a stab at understanding the other person and responds at this 'common sense' level. If mistakes are made, they are cleared up as the dialogue unfolds.

The method of addressing the data, described here, is a similar process. The researcher is exploring a range of meanings in what is offered to him in the form of text. The *rigor* of the process is *the attempt at being exhaustive of possible meanings*. Nor is the *source* of such meanings particularly limited. The skilled researcher may draw on psychology, sociology, literature, poetry, theology, popular culture and so on in his search for meanings for the text in front of him. In this sense, that analysis is akin to *literary criticism*. And, after all, the text in front of the research is just another form of text and, as we have seen, might more interestingly be viewed as a form of fiction. And just as, presumably, no one still attempts to decide what 'Shakespeare really meant', nor need the researcher, necessarily try to discern what the interviewee really meant.

This style of analysis would not aim at any sort of consensus. There need not be (though there could be) comparisons of transcripts. Indeed, the analysis could be carried out on a single transcript. Alternatively, as is the case when novels are compared and contrasted, two or three transcripts could be examined together. There would, however, be no grouping together of ideas nor any search for categories.

The process described here would lead to 'messy' or 'fuzzy' findings. The researcher could not (and would not want to) generalize from his or her findings. Those findings would be in the form of detailed commentaries and narratives.

It is not suggested that this might or should become a principle method of qualitative analysis but merely to head in another direction. At the start of this section, it was suggested that qualitative analysis has become, necessarily, reductionist. This section has outlined one way of thinking about doing qualitative research differently. More work will have to be done and more thinking will have to take place about various ways of operationalising the ideas described here. It is hoped, however, that the section will spark some discussion and lead to some further thinking about how best to work with textual data generated in a qualitative study.

Various questions may be raised at once. How *many* interpretations might a research make of any given text? Are *all* interpretations appropriate or should the researcher have to *justify* his or her interpretations? Should the respondent be brought into the process of interpretation - in much the same way as a poet may or may not be brought into a discussion about his or her poems? Should the idea of searching for the respondent's 'real meaning' be lost entirely or could various methods of textual analysis be combined? How long would it take to complete a given piece of research and - perhaps most important of all in the current climate - would researchers using this approach be awarded researcher funding? It remains to be seen.

All sorts of objections may be raised to this approach. First, is the idea that we are somehow divorcing a transcript of a person's interview from what that person 'meant' during that interview. This objection, it is claimed, is dealt with, above, via the suggestion that any such search for 'real' meaning is an illusion. Second, the objection may be made that such an approach is entirely subjective and that is could lead to a sort of 'research anarchy'. It is fully acknowledged that the approach is entirely subjective and that different researchers would offer different sets of interpretations of textual datasets. This, however, is viewed as a *strength* of the process in much the same way as different interpretations of a piece of music or a play may be welcomed. There is, arguably, no definitive interpretation of a piece of music: neither is there a definitive interpretation of what an interview transcript means.

Another objection may be that this represents a form of 'flabby relativism' - that all views are valid and no one view is any better or worse than any other. This objection may be met by the suggestion that the form of interpretation offered here might *supplement* other forms of qualitative analysis. It is not a question of *this* method *replacing* others but simply a question of the method offering another perspective. It seems possible to imagine a qualitative researcher first analyzing a text by the methods described in the early part of this section, followed by a second analysis using the method offered here.

A related objection might be that 'just because we cannot reach a absolute understanding of what another person means, does not mean that we should abandon all attempts at trying'. In other words, the qualitative researcher might want to argue that we should at least attempt to understand what another person is saying to us. This is, of course, a valid point but one that is missing the *purpose* of the type of analysis proposed here. The aim, as has been suggested, is not to understand the respondent's point of view but to explore interview transcripts from another perspective. Again, it might be suggested that both of the types of approaches alluded to in this section could be used in data analysis.

A third objection may be the question: 'what's the point?' The point, perhaps, is to use text to *generate ideas*, to offer new insights by imaginatively exploring textual data from a variety of points of views. The approach is offered, not in any sense as *the* way of approaching textual data but rather in the spirit that this could be *another* way of exploring meaning systems, ideas and utterances in social science research.

A final objection, in this short list, might be the question 'how could it be done?' It has to be admitted that further work would have to be done to develop a *method* of analysis of this sort. The aim of this section has been to identify a different approach to the handling of textual data in qualitative research and, perhaps, to redress the balance a little. The researcher who used this approach would have to be flexible, well read, open minded and prepared to make all sorts of 'leaps in the dark'. The outcomes would be unpredictable and the 'findings' from such a study would have a different status to those from more traditional studies. The gains, however, might be in helping us, however obliquely, to more fully understand the human condition.

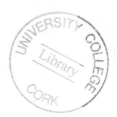

4 The findings

The presentation of the findings follows, as perceived by the researcher, a logical, but an arguably arbitrary order. Indeed, it has been pointed out that the reporting of qualitative data confronts the researcher with a difficult problem, as there is no well codified, generally accepted protocol as to how these findings can be best communicated (Munhall and Oliver 1986).

First, the unique features of working in an acute psychiatric environment are described. The roles and skills of the nurses are then described and analysed, followed by a description and analysis of how these are influenced by a number of factors. Finally, a description and analysis of the relationship that nurses have with other health professionals is offered.

Working with a small sample necessitated the need for anonymity and confidentiality. None of the respondents will therefore be referred to by grade or, in the case of the other health professionals, by discipline. This has resulted in losing some of the richness of the data.

Setting the scene

As a way of introducing the clinical environment, it may be useful to identify what the respondents thought the unique features of working in an acute psychiatric unit are, and the special skills and qualities that are required.

Nurses identified the spontaneity, the fluidity, the variety, and the daily challenge to respond quickly as the unique features. Forming relationships with "psychotic" people formed part of that challenge. Indeed, spending time, being available over 24 hours, or just being there was considered by nurses to be the main reason for their existence in that environment.

Non nurse respondents also commented on the nurses' opportunities to develop relationships. In addition they saw nurses as the hosts, the ambassadors, making patients feel welcome and comfortable.

There was general agreement that nursing in this environment required special skills and qualities. Working under pressure a lot of the time was one of those qualities. One respondent also observed that:

> a nurse has to be fairly sure of her own skills in dealing with people in an acute environment...

Reference was made by non nurse respondents to the intensity of working in an acute unit, and the many anxieties that nurses are exposed to and needed to contain. That, observed one, required a lot of inner stability.

Finally, all respondents singled out one particular ability that stood out from all others, namely the ability to deal with potential and actual disturbances, volatile situations, and threatening and violent behaviours. Nurses apparently had these skills, mainly because of the frequent occurrences on the wards:

> ...you have special skills, things like giving space...

> ...you need specific skills of sitting down, calming somebody who is highly disturbed...

> ...to deal with violent situations, that's the most frightening of all, how to deal with that requires tremendous skill...

The role of the nurse

The data seemed to suggest that nurses in this setting performed a wide range of roles, which contained elements of that of caretaker, role-model, policeman, container, custodian, arbitrator, mediator, informer, co-ordinator, manager, and administrator, but with few suggestions of that of an autonomous, independent therapeutic agent.

Indeed, nurses referred to themselves as "jack of all trades", although as one nurse emphasised "not necessarily master of none", indicating that dealing with psychotic behaviour was what she "mastered".

Non nurse respondents also perceived nurses as "skilled generalists", involved in caring rather than treatment, with a certain level of competency in quite a few areas. One stressed that nurses should be jack of all trades, but they need to specialise in one or two skills, if, as he suggested, they did not want to remain "dogsbodies" all their lives. The term "dogsbody", used by this respondent, revealed quite an derogatory attitude towards nurses.

Others described nurses as being at the "coalface, the prime movers". This was considered by both nurse and non nurse respondents to be the unique role of the nurse:

> you're the on site main person, being there, the parent or call it whatever you want... the fact that somebody is available over 24 hours...they (patients) don't make an appointment to see you.

Concern was expressed about the often conflicting roles, especially that of counsellor and manager. This led one non nurse respondent to comment that certain things needed to be done by other people, in different places.

The nurse as mediator, between patients and other disciplines, but also between patients themselves, was highlighted by several respondents:

> you're sort of stuck in the middle...

> nurses have to be around to manage disruptive behaviour, difficulties between patients.

Managing the environment, providing a physical and psychological structure, was also highlighted as an important component of the nurse's role:

> my job is to provide an environment for patients to conductively receive care, appropriate to their needs, as safely and effectively as we can...it isn't just about patient care, it's about keeping the place ticking over, the environment needs to be managed.

Respondents were divided in their perceptions whether nurses were moving from being custodians to becoming therapeutic agents. Being a custodian was associated by some with observing and providing care to people who were admitted on sections of the 1983 Mental Health Act:

> our job is to keep patients in hospital; for example, sectioning a patient results in observation...so that's a custodial role.

Others acknowledged the fine balance between both concepts, and recognised that custodial care can, or should be therapeutic:

> there are times that you have to step in, to be a custodian when for example you're secluding others or individuals themselves, although you can say that you're also a therapeutic agent by doing that.

> ...in some cases custody is therapeutic. People like boundaries to make them feel safe...it reduces their anxiety.

Others went further, and suggested that it would be neglectful of a nurse to say they're just therapists, arguing that if nurses were not there to contain disturbed patients, then sitting down, having long therapy sessions would not be a substitute at all. It was also recognised that the more therapeutic skills a nurse possessed, for example establishing rapport and trust, the less likely it would be that you would be a custodian.

Custody then was associated with managing the environment, managing people, and making use of interpersonal skills.

Therapeutic skills

The skills that respondents perceived nurses to use, and having therapeutic value, have been categorised as interpersonal skills, care related skills, organisational skills, custodial skills. In addition, a number of skills have been categorised under the heading "miscellaneous".

Respondents found it difficult to describe what they understood by "therapeutic skills", and often responded with:

...it depends what you mean by therapeutic work.

One nurse suggested that you could be engaged in therapeutic work when:

you're walking with someone to the toilet, a patient may be saying something to you, so in that sense it's difficult to quantify.

A non nurse respondent referred to the notion of providing structure in one's work:

to try to be specific when you see a patient and for how long.

Another non nurse respondent suggested that it was not a question of possessing skills, but having personal qualities that were an integral part of oneself. She argued therefore that:

I cannot give my skills away, I would be giving something of myself away...

Interpersonal skills

Nurses identified a range of interpersonal skills that could be best described as a continuum of basic communication skills to the more counselling oriented skills.

Listening was mentioned most frequently in this context, and this ran along the dimension of "being a soundingboard", to attempting to understand and help patients make sense of their experiences. Active listening skills such as reflecting, paraphrasing and clarifying were mentioned. In addition, nurses identified a number of counselling strategies, such as helping patients focus on their problems, setting mutual goals, and pointing out alternatives. Conditions deemed necessary for effective interaction, such as empathy, warmth and understanding were also referred to. Some used particular frameworks in their interactions, for example Transactional Analysis (Berne 1964) and Six Category Intervention Analysis (Heron 1990).

Self awareness, awareness of transference, role modelling and a number of non verbal communication skills, especially touch, were mentioned by a minority of nurses.

Nurses often referred to personal qualities rather than skills, such as being adaptable, flexible, having patience, a sense of humour, and a high degree of tolerance:

> You have to be quite strong from a psychological point of view in so far as being able to take on board a lot of the aggression and the grief, but not in destructive way to yourself.

Non nurse respondents identified a similar range of skills and qualities, with again the emphasis on active listening skills. Although empathy was considered important, one respondent stressed that it was the nurse's ability to be able to contain patients' anxieties, without being pushed into action, that was the most difficult part for nurses to master. Even so, talking people through a crisis and settling down psychotic patients after an admission were seen as important interpersonal skills to have.

The way nurses used touch to comfort patients was reflected upon by one respondent:

> When to do it, and when not to do it...with some people it would feel quite persecuting or seductive or exciting...or to balance it up.
> There may be a bit of misinterpretation, but on the whole it would be better to do it than not to do it.

This respondent added that she did not consider it appropriate for her to be engaged in that activity.

The notion of providing time and space was difficult to translate into a skill, however that seemed to contain the essence of what the respondents identified in relation to their interpersonal skills and qualities. One non nurse respondent talked about patients getting a lot of help from the "simple humanity" that some nurses showed, referring to giving time and listening to patients. This seemed to correspond with an observation by a nurse, which appeared to capture the essence:

> It's about giving people time to express their hopes and fears, their worries about what happens here, to generally give them information what's happening, what could be organised, the how and when of the system.

Closely linked to these interpersonal skills was the development of trusting relationships, which nurses attempted, but not always managed to establish with patients. This one-to-one relationship was thought possible within a system of primary nursing. Non nurse respondents also identified a high demand in this setting for individual work with patients. For them, this provided nurses with opportunities to "get to know the patients quite well." Indeed, through this relationship patients disclosed sensitive issues:

> Those things are often disclosed to nurse, not to anyone else. That's due to the nurse's skill in establishing rapport, making it safe to disclose those skeletons in people's cupboards.

An important aspect of the nurse's interpersonal skills was their ability to respond to potential and actual aggressive and violent situations. This was perceived by both respondents as an almost exclusive skill of nurses. Anger management, containing violence and "real craziness" were seen to be the domain of nursing practice:

> If I had a patient who I was really worried about being violent, I would be much happier if there was a nurse around, because they do know, they can be very good when somebody may get out of hand, at what level to intervene...

This was either because nurses had the interpersonal skills to defuse the situation, or the perceived ability and authority to physically remove a person.

Care related skills

These could be categorised as skills within the framework of the nursing process. Observation skills were mentioned quite frequently, and this related to skills of observing the behaviours and interactions of patients, and generally what goes on the ward, mainly with the idea to:

> look for clues, gain an awareness, an understanding.

Closely related to the skills of observation were the skills of assessing people's mental and physical state, and their level of functioning, with a view to develop plans of action and interventions.

It was interesting to note that only non nurse respondents mentioned the nurse's skills to provide practical and physical support, to help patients with self care:

> simple day to day activities, bathing etc., the sort of thing mothers do for their children... helping patients who need a lot of help when they first come in...

although it could be argued that nurses did not perceive these to be therapeutic skills.

Organisational skills

In contrast to nurses, non nurse respondents talked at length about the importance of the ability of nurses to organise and manage the environment, patients and themselves. Nurses were seen as providing not only a physical and psychological structure, but also ensured that the patient's care was structured and co-ordinated:

> getting to things on time, getting them to organise themselves, looking after themselves, care for themselves is a major part of inpatient psychiatric nursing...

In addition, they highlighted the importance for nurses to co-ordinate treatments, investigations, and the necessary paperwork. Working with, liaising and being part of a multi-disciplinary team were also perceived to be relevant skills to have.

Custodial skills

Physical and psychological containment was another area that was highlighted more by non nurses than nurses. Skills relating to the provision of safety and protection, the containment of disturbed patients and "parenting operations" were perceived to be the expertise of nurses:

> ...make them feel safe, they've been out of control, they need some containment...boundaries got to be reinforced.

> ...stopping them escaping, there's a lot of work in that, especially in this environment, where it is easy for patients to disappear.

Miscellaneous

Finally, a range of other skills were alluded to briefly by all the respondents, such as skills relating to behaviour therapy, cognitive therapy, and leading patient groups. In addition, teaching, education, giving advice and providing information about:

> medication, their illness, the implications of the diagnosis, how to cope, info about what's happening to them, telling them about the Unit...

were highlighted.

Pharmacological knowledge, skills in relation to the administration of medication, knowledge about a range of symptoms and illnesses, and an understanding of the "system" were also identified.

Finally, mention was made of nurses' abilities, or potential abilities to work with relatives and carers of patients.

Some general comments on skills

Nurses commented that they needed to have a wide range of skills:

> given that our clientele is so vast, from mild disorders to severe
> levels of mental illness...

but suggested that they were better skilled with "psychotic" people, rather than people with "anxiety". Attempts were made by ward managers to look at specific skills and experiences of nurses, for example grief work, before deciding on a primary nurse for patients.

Asked whether they knew they were effective in their employment of various skills, nurses suggested that it was difficult to measure, and that there were too many factors:

> I've no idea how you could measure it...I can go through an
> intervention, but I don't know at the end of six months care and
> say it's because this and this approach. It's not that structured, but
> that's not to demean the work and say it doesn't make a difference.

Non nurses commented on the enormous differences in nurses' abilities, with some very traditional medically oriented nurses, other who would make good psychotherapists, and some falling in between.

Finally, both respondents suggested that skills are not necessarily learned in training, but had to do with confidence, empowerment, experience, trial and error, personal maturity and a common sense approach:

> people who do well usually have a certain personal
> sophistication...

Deficiencies, developments and boundaries

A range of skills and qualities have been identified and described. Although counselling and establishing relationships were seen as important components of the nurses' work, a number of the respondents felt that those skills could be further developed. In addition, nurses identified a need to develop more in-depth skills in behavioural interventions, skills in relation to working with people with alcohol and drug problems, because of an increase in admissions in this area, skills dealing with bereavement, and skills in relation to working with adolescents and people with anorexia nervosa. These areas were then referred on to other disciplines. Some saw this as a strength because:

> it would be arrogant to think we could do everything ourselves.

It was recognised that those referrals were appropriate when "it required in-depth work" and when "more specialists skills" were needed. Nurses recognised their limitations in those areas, but also seemed to suggest that certain skills and knowledge belong to particular disciplines, for example housing and finance to social workers, living skills assessment and implementation to occupational therapists, while bereavement counselling and behavioural programmes were seen to belong to the psychologist's domain. It is interesting to note that the psychiatrist's domain was not mentioned.

Non nurse respondents identified other areas in which they felt nurses could develop their skills, for example working with families and relatives. However, two skills in particular were highlighted: group work skills and assertiveness skills.

The deficiency in group work skills seemed to be cause for concern:

> I've been involved in the morning group...nursing staff find that terribly difficult, because they haven't had any training in groups...some do, they have a much better idea.

> They often don't know what to do...it's quite tempting to be directive...or not saying anything at all...I've felt so frustrated, nobody else is helping me.

These may have been assumptions, or expectations, regarding responsibilities for leading those groups. This was expressed by one non nurse respondent, who:

often feels very uncomfortable to take the lead...I attend one morning a week and the nurses look to me as the leader.

Others however pointed out that nurses are not in a position to lead:

Yes, nurses can run groups and they can be very good, but sometimes you need somebody who's trained and then nurses can be co-workers.

Non nurse respondents also expressed concern about the lack of assertiveness and self confidence among nurses. Those areas will be described under the category "Influencing care and treatment".

A variety of explanations were proposed by the respondents why nurses lacked certain skills. These ranged from lack of preparation in nurse education, the diversity of problems that nurses were faced with on the ward, to lack of experience and opportunities, and the personality of the nurse.

Factors influencing the employment of skills

This area generated a considerable quantity of data. It could be argued that this was the most important issued on the respondents' minds. However, by expressing their concerns to the researcher, they may have anticipated to influence - indirectly - policies and practices on the ward, once the outcome of the study had been made available. Alternatively, they may have felt an opportunity to offload their concerns and frustrations to a non-judgmental listener. Finally, it simply may have been that there were that many constraints that hindered nurses from using their skills and potential.

A range of factors influences whether nurses felt, or were able to use their skills. These factors appeared to relate to environmental, organisational, managerial, personal and administrative aspects, although these seemed often interlinked. Time, interruptions and having no control were the continuous threads running through these various aspects.

Responses from nurses suggested that they continuously have to establish how to make the best use of their available time. Administrative duties, servicing others took priority over therapeutic activities. As one nurse explained:

> ...sometimes you know somebody is in tears, who needs to speak to someone, and you've got a ward round to go to, write an account of how 14 patients spent the morning...Dividing your time, that can be difficult.

Responding to senior management and doing administrative work interfered with therapeutic work, which nurses seemed to value more:

> I was seeing somebody the other day whom I knew had been upset...I had been speaking to her for about 20 minutes and was interrupted by the ward clerk: "(Senior nurse manager) wants to see you". "Cannot, I'm busy now". "It's urgent". So you drop all tools, leave patient with her feelings...Establishment figures have a higher priority than talking to a distressed client.

> ...person with most experience spends least time with patients...you don't get paid for being a good clinician.

Porter (1993), drawing on the work of Strauss et al (1981), suggests that rules relating to order are far more common and specific. Procedures around for example incidents and abscondments merit considerable attention, while there are no prescriptive rules relating to communicating and interacting with patients. As a result, he concludes, a nurse is likely to get into trouble for failures in maintenance of order, rather than for failures in therapy.

Clinical grading further influenced the amount of time a nurse spends on administration:

> As a ward manager you sit in the office, doing an off-duty...doing silly things like answering the telephone, somebody else could do that, take messages...I trained to be a nurse.

The office became the focal point for a variety of interactions, including interactions between nurses and patients:

most of my time is in the office...patients come to the office, there's often a queue waiting to see you...so your contact is more than you think...although it is very short, very quick.

if you're the only qualified staff on...you can spend 90% of the time in the office, seeing to this and that.

Non nurse respondents also commented on the amount of time that nurses spend on administrative and clerical duties, which kept them away from patients. One suggested that this was a recent development:

...administrative stuff, isn't particularly therapeutic...I think trained nurses don't get that much time to get out of the office to spend more time with the patients at all.

...in the past, there was more time to talk to patients, you very seldom get the trained nurse to go to a patient to chat to them, unless the patient comes to the office.

Not all nurses perceived the managerial aspects of their role as negative. Some regarded it as a positive step, a move forward in developing management skills.

The nature of the environment, and the admission and discharge policies and practices also influenced the way nurses employed their skills. The data suggested that nurses had virtually no control over the wide and varying range of admissions. This diversity was considered to be a major constraint:

We tend to take whatever comes through the door...a broad spectrum...all and sundry...you cannot refuse.

...that's the problem, given that we're a hospital that covers a catchment area, you cannot pick or choose the problems that your clients come in with.

Turner-Crowson (1993) identifies a number of common concerns of clients and families in relation to hospital admissions, that influences the way the mental health nurse functions. She supports the notion that mental health nurses have a contribution to make in helping to change the practice of inappropriate admissions, overcrowding, rundown units, little meaningful activities, insensitive, stultifying and disabling treatments, and a lack of alternatives to hospital admissions.

In addition, the high turnover of patients was considered to be an influencing factor:

> the acute side of their illness is dealt with as much as possible, then they're discharged.

A number of reports have raised this issue among a range of other concerns (M.H.A.C. 1993; D.O.H. 1994b; Royal College of Psychiatrists 1994), some of which were alluded to earlier. Other areas identified relate to patient mix, in terms of age and levels of disturbance, inadequate staffing levels, leading to controlling rather than therapeutic practices, and the mainly administrative duties of senior staff. The mental health nursing review (D.O.H. 1994a) found that many nurses considered that the units attached to District General Hospitals (D.G.H.'s) had serious deficiencies as a therapeutic setting, and argue for an urgent review of the therapeutic suitability of these mental health units. This brings in to question the place and function of the acute psychiatric unit, and the place and function of the nurse within it, in mental health care provision. Crisis care can be provided in different forms and in different settings, at apparently similar costs, as recent studies have demonstrated (Dean and Gadd 1990; Marks et al 1994; Knapp et al 1994).

One nurse summed it up as follows:

> You've got a whole load of patients, with a wide range of disturbances...they're all under one roof...severe levels of anxiety, psychosis, lack of insight, trust, high levels of depression, high risk of suicide, levels of paranoia...

This is supported by a non nurse respondent who used a warfare metaphor to sum up the situation:

> There must sometimes be a bombardment of an enormous range of needs.

Although some took this situation as given, others were more concerned:

> I don't think it's good to have such a vast range of conditions...the range here is too great...the stay for a lot of people is more traumatic than their illness.

The diversity of needs and the levels of disturbances in turn then appeared to lead to reactive and interrupted use of their skills. Indeed, interruptions were high on the respondents' minds:

> The whole nature of the work is ad hoc, dealing with things as they crop up, rather than planning for it.
> I'd like to be able to sit down with patients in need...but I don't get the opportunity to sit down without being interrupted...you cannot let a colleague get beaten up, when they shout, you go. That happens on a regular basis...that's been my experience, also on other acute settings I've worked in. I don't think it should be.

Nurses seemed to value individualised care, and perceived the establishment of relationships with patients as important, but felt unable to do so:

> Sometimes it takes a lot to establish a relationship with a patient, it may be at a crucial point, something happens, you may be taken away, it takes a lot to get back.

> There's never continuity, beginning and terminating interactions appropriately rarely occurs.

Respondents indicate that all these problems could be overcome, if only nurses had the time. "Time" continuously returned as one of the most important factors. Nurses' responses to the question how much time they did spend in direct patient contact however varied from "very little" to "most of the day", with various grades in-between. The majority of non nurse respondents felt they were not in a position to comment on this issue, although some suggested that the clinical grade of nurse had a direct relationship to the time spent with patients. Others proposed that the interest and willingness of nurses themselves to interact were influencing factors.

One nurse described the element of time in this manner:

> Time is the factor. In order to come across to somebody, they have to know that you're willing to give them your time, and you got to give them this time beforehand, so they can build up this psychological safety, so they can offload and talk to you...all you are able to do is glance around in the morning, chat to them over the trolley and if there's a catastrophe spend ten minutes with them.

The perceived lack of time also led to an inability to employ any therapeutic intervention in any great depth:

> I am very interested in cognitive therapy and redressing people's negative thoughts; you try and do it in passing, but in no way can you get it across in any meaningful structured way in this situation.

Brief counselling and group work were also mentioned in this context. One nurse commented that interventions in this acute environment could only take place at an elementary level anyway, because of the "level of functioning of acute patients".

Non nurse respondents expressed similar observations regarding the unstructured nature and its affect on nurses' ability to use their skills:

> it seems a bit hit and miss...it depends how busy the ward is, but also the particular interest of the nurse, or the wishes of the patients.

Indeed, it was pointed out by one non nurse respondent that it was only possible to do any therapeutic work if patients were receptive to it.

Personal tolerance and the lack of adequate support and supervision was another area that respondents identified as influencing the effective employment of their skills:

> How much can one person take "on board" and use (skills) positively without supervision and adequate time and support.

60

A non nurse respondent referred to the anxieties that patients were communicating, which, she suggested, were very difficult to know what to do with:

> I think the fear that one may not be able to bear it, that it will get inside you, disturb you, all those things get in the way...nurses aren't helped nearly enough to understand the sorts of feelings, the powerful processes that inevitably go on...they protect themselves with the structure of the job, the nursing duties they have to carry out are protective to the staff...

Ferguson (1992) indicated that supervision arrangements in in-patient settings were poorly developed. Equally, the mental health nursing review's report (D.O.H. 1994a) found that adequate clinical supervision is not yet the norm for the majority of mental health nurses, although the report stresses that there are notable exceptions. Faugier (1994), among others, point out that clinical supervision in mental health nursing is crucial to its development, and one may add, to its survival. She compares clinical supervision with miners' pit-head time, in which miners had the right to wash off grime from the job in the employer's time. Faugier (1994) proposes "pit-head time for those who work at the coal face of emotional distress, disease, death, loss and confusion (p.65)". The mental health nursing review (D.O.H. 1994) identifies some groundrules for this "pit-head time".

Without exception, all respondents identified the staffing levels and the skill mix as important factors that influenced the way nurses performed their roles and used their skills. This of course cannot be separated from the factors that have been identified earlier, such as time, interruptions, supervision and the ad hoc nature of their work.

Nurses reported that, on average, two qualified nurses were on duty per shift, supported by a number of unqualified staff in the form of nursing assistants and health care assistants (HCA's), providing nursing care for a maximum of 24 patients:

> ...if you want to plan, it may happen, but you cannot always be consistent...

...two qualified staff per shift, one is in the ward round, the other doesn't have the time.

...there is a certain amount you can do, and the rest, probably 2 unqualified, who are observing patients who need close observation...there isn't the time to do things therapeutically that we could do.

Concern was expressed not only about the increasing number of HCA's on the ward, but also about their limited abilities, and its effect on both the quality of patient care and the level of support they require:

It seems they need more support than maybe some of our clients.

This in turn led to tensions and frustrations among qualified staff:

We are the parrots in the office...HCA's are on the ward, hardly knowing how to deal with situations, problems...it's not fair on them, not fair on qualified staff. You end up overburdened, frustrated, overworked, often venting that frustration on them (HCA's).

These responses seem to confirm the results of White's (1991) Delphi study, which suggested that nurses were concerned, and thought it undesirable, that their work would consist predominantly of supervising H.C.A.'s. Nurses in White's study also predicted, and again thought this to be undesirable, that patients' therapeutic contact time would be mainly with junior staff and H.C.A.'s.

Finally, the respondents identified a range of other factors that influenced the way nurses were able to employ their skills. These were for example chemotherapeutic factors: "if people are very, very overmedicated"; environmental factors: "nurses do not have the luxury of having their own room"; deep seated institutional factors: "let's sit down and have coffee and deal with patients at a certain time" and hierarchical managerial factors: "the system, the nature of the people in charge, it's partly about power".

The inability to use one's skills to their full potential led to a variety of responses. Frustration, tension, and in the end, people giving up and leaving:

> You've got to work under high levels of pressure and tension, with less and less staff...you've go to be seen to be coping...

> I've known staff who have left because they cannot do what they want to do.

Bamber (1988) found that in one hospital there was a wastage rate of 53% a year among psychiatric nurses. Poor management and staff relations, lack of resources, poor pay, and a dislike of the hospital culture were given as reasons for leaving. Leavers apparently had higher stress levels and were more dissatisfied.

Brown et al (1994) examined stress levels among community psychiatric nurses and ward based psychiatric nurses. Using the Maslach Burnout Inventory (Maslach and Jackson 1986), they found that, although both groups scored moderate to high on emotional exhaustion, ward based nurses scored significantly higher on depersonalisation, which seems to indicate that these nurses were experiencing more alienation and lack of empathy towards clients than community psychiatric nurses. In addition, ward based nurses also experienced high levels of burn out in personal accomplishment and feelings of futility at work, suggesting greater levels of frustration and hopelessness. In spite of this however, both groups seemed satisfied with their jobs.

Working with other health professionals

Respondents suggested that care and treatment in this acute psychiatric environment was delivered by various different health professionals, working within a multi-disciplinary framework. This section describes and analyses the relationship between nurses and those other disciplines, and the position of nurses in that multi-disciplinary framework. These relationships and the position of nurses in the multi-disciplinary team again influenced the way nurses employed their skills.

Responses from nurses suggested that they felt their job was in some ways harder and less rewarding:

> We take people when they're at their worst.

implying perhaps that others may have an easier and more fulfilling role to play. Indeed, one non nurse respondent pointed out that she only got involved when patients were "getting better". There may have been a hint of resentment among nurses:

> You can say that our best patients attend Occupational Therapy, so they get off lightly.

This resentment grew stronger when nurses were called upon to deal with disruptive patients or volatile situations:

> It's a standing joke...they call for a nurse...because a nurse can give an injection... or model a calm approach.

Dealing with those situations was seen by other disciplines to fall within the domain of the nurse, although nurses themselves seemed to perceive it as doing someone else's dirty work.

Nurses pointed out that their position was very different, mainly because they were there all the time, providing care 24 hours a day. This meant that they saw the "whole picture" rather than a "snapshot". They could not be selective in their choice of patient:

> We take all and sundry, whatever comes through the door.

The picture of the nurse as generalist emerged, mopping up, assisting others, but lacking a clear identity of what they should be doing themselves. A non nurse respondent described it in this way:

> (Nurses) feel that they do the everyday muck, they are there all the time, not as specialists as the doctor, the occupational therapist, the community psychiatric nurse or the social worker...maybe because of the general, not specific...they tend to do everything else, but not the basic nursing.

Responses from non nurse respondents suggested that they had a better sense of their own identity and were much clearer about their specialist skills:

> We start out from a more secure standpoint in terms of our identity.

> I would not expect them (nurses) to be as effective at designing cognitive behavioural interventions as I am.

However, one non nurse respondent pointed out that nurses could do exactly the same therapeutic work, if they had the time and the physical space available to them.

This division between the generalist nurse and the specialist other professional appeared to lead to a division of labour in which nurses were considered as assisting these other professionals in the performance of their work Nurses' were relied upon to make sure patients turned up for therapeutic activities, during which time the nurses may function as co-therapists in for example group work. Nurses informed other disciplines about patient behaviours; these other disciplines then designed treatment programmes for nurse to implement.

Although this could be construed as complementing each other's roles and skills, it seemed to lead to conflict, resentment, rivalry and competition about where and by whom certain therapeutic activities ought to be carried out. This was reflected by a non nurse respondent who pointed out that:

everybody likes to do a bit of counselling...sometimes you forget what your role is...it's important to stick to your role...if it's all enmeshed, then you're getting nowhere.

Another non nurse respondent attempted to put herself in the position of nurses and suggested that nurses may think that:

What do they (other disciplines) have to offer, we've trained in anxiety management, we've trained in counselling, we've trained in activities of daily living etc...

adding that there was no way that nurses could have the training of everyone and be expected to take over, although she felt that some did have that expectation. She suspected a sense of antagonism:

interprofessional rivalry and suspicion...the idea of coming in to do the glory bit instead of doing the hands on implementation, which leads to (nurses) sabotaging it by the actual way of putting it (programme) into practice.

Influencing care and treatment

Nurses varied in their responses about the influence they thought they had in the decision making process in relation to patient care and treatment within the multi-disciplinary team. This influence was mainly based on the notion that they spent most time with the patients, which was considered an advantage they had over other professionals.

Responses then varied from "very significant", because of their understanding and knowledge of the patients, to "quite influential" and "fairly influential" because they felt they were being listened to. Others were less certain:

you can be overruled...but overall, I think we have an influence. I hope we do...sometimes I feel it is taken on board...other times they tend to dismiss you.

Non nurse respondents were less convincing about the influence that nurses had, especially in relation to influencing consultants. The latter were seen to have a "skewed" influence over the thinking in the team, whereas:

> I often feel nurses have a much better feel for the patients...if I was a nurse I would get furious, the way doctors just take over, think they know best.

There appeared to be an attempt to recognise nurses as equal partners, but as one non nurse respondent pointed out:

> they have to make their voice heard, it's no good being there as a member and having to be asked: "Well, what do you think?" "Oh, she's all right" You don't want that kind of thing...we want some sort of input..."I've something to contribute. I'm a professional like you, and you should listen to me"...So often nurses have taken a backward seat, you have to encourage them to come forward, maybe they've been kept in that role by the hierarchy.

The hierarchical nursing structure was indeed used as a possible explanation:

> It seems to be a lack of a sense of power very often...to challenge the consultant...very often nurses haven't got that, they're just the nurses and that's awful.

The same respondent argued however that nurses must take some of the blame for accepting their subordinate role:

> It's their fault too...I often sit there thinking "Hell, you know, they're with them (patients) all the time".

This lack of assertiveness presented itself very strongly, especially among the non nurse respondents. Some nurses recognised this:

> it takes a very assertive nurse to get her voice heard.

67

The power of the medical profession was given as an explanation. Multi-disciplinary teams were considered by most respondents to be "consultant-dominated":

> It depends how much input they let you have...if he's pleasant, he'll listen, if he's ignorant, he rules, only him.

Suggestions were made that nurses were influenced by the personality of the consultant, and felt intimidated. One non nurse respondent pointed out that in some cases it did not really matter what anybody else said. In those circumstances however it was an advantage to be any professional but a nurse:

> It would be easier for me to argue with the doctor...a doctor cannot tell me what to do.

implying that doctors were in a position to tell nurses what to do, which may stem from the traditional hierarchical doctor-nurse relationship.

The data then seemed to suggest that there was a discrepancy in perception between nurse and non nurse respondents in relation to the influence that nurses have in patient care. Levels of experience, feelings of adequacy and confidence, hierarchical structures, conflicting ideologies, were identified as possible explanations for nurses' lack of assertiveness in the multi-disciplinary team.

On the basis of the data presented the following differentiation between nurses and other disciplines is proposed.

Nurses:	Other Disciplines:
* generalist "dogsbody"	* specialist
* take all and sundry	* selective
* when patients are "at worst"	* when patients get better
* see whole picture	* snapshot

*	being in the front-line	*	behind the scene
*	being there "24 hours"	*	sporadic
*	"as things happen"	*	by appointment
*	data-collectors "parrots"	*	designers
*	implementors	*	evaluators
*	passive	*	assertive
*	assistants/co-workers	*	primary therapists
*	care	*	treatment
*	vague role definition	*	clear identity
*	little influence	*	more influential
*	"ad hoc" intervention	*	structured intervention
*	co-ordinators		
*	administrators	*	therapists

A similar trend was reported by Ward (1993). He expressed concern that in the USA the involvement of psychiatric nurses focused on providing other professions with the information they require to carry out their therapy roles, which means that therapeutic input is provided by other health care professionals. It seems that nurses have now become handmaidens of all other health care personnel.

5 Discussion of the findings

In this chapter the findings of the study are discussed, with the aim of drawing together some of the themes and issues that were highlighted in the previous chapter, and linking those with the prescribed and described literature.

The findings suggested that first level nurses in this acute psychiatric admission environment performed a wide range of different roles. Within these roles they employed a number of therapeutic skills and personal qualities to meet the many demands that they faced. Although there was some evidence to suggest that nurses ascribed to the idea of developing therapeutic relationships with the patients, and indeed expressed that they attempted to base their work on humanistic principles, the findings suggested that they had only limited opportunities to develop those relationships.

There was a lack of clarity as to what was understood by the term "therapeutic". A suggestion was made that any interaction could potentially be therapeutic, but this did not seem to be what Strupp (1986) referred to as a systematic use of human relationships to effect change.

The therapeutic role prescribed in the literature did not seem to be realised in practice. Clarke (1988) has argued that nurses may be unwilling or unable to accept a therapeutic role for themselves in relation to other disciplines, and suggested that nurses may contribute to the preservation of the existing system.

The emphasis of the nurses' work seemed to be mainly on managing the environment and the patients, other nurses and themselves within it. Managing appeared to have a care-taking and controlling character, focusing on patient behaviours, rather than focusing on the facilitation of recovery and change. "Keeping the place ticking over" meant creating ward order, maintaining the safety of staff and patients, and ensuring that patients arrived on time for their therapeutic activities. The orientation in their work seemed based on paternalistic principles.

Nolan (1993) has suggested that different professional groups have different beliefs about what they do. In this study nurses were seen as skilled generalists by the other disciplines, with limited skills in a variety of areas, but also there to assist them in the performance of their role. This consisted in for example collecting information about patients, taking patients to therapeutic activities, and performing a range of co-ordinating and administrative activities. Nurses however were valued by the other professionals for their skills and qualities in managing disturbances, aggression and violence.

Other disciplines considered themselves to be more specialist practitioners, and seemed to have a clearer identity about their role than nurses had. There were skills that the different professional groups shared with each other, for example counselling and group work skills. These overlapping areas gave also rise to resentment, jealousy and suspicion, all professionals claiming expertise and protecting their vested interests.

Applying Bunch's (1985) structural requirements to the findings of this study, a suggestion could be made that the institutional requirements often took precedence over the professional and clinical requirements. The roles and skills that nurses performed were, it seemed, determined by the organisational structures, ideologies, practices and policies over which nurses seemed to have, or exercised little control. Although nurses valued and attempted to develop therapeutic relationships with the patients, they felt unable to establish these, being hindered by these factors, but also by the perceived low staffing levels. This resulted in unsystematic, unstructured, ad hoc, often interrupted and mainly reactive and controlling practices. Cormack (1983) has pointed out that the unstructured nature of nurses' work may be a valuable form of unsystematic and unrecognised therapy. Indeed, nurses attached a great deal of value to the importance of spending time with and giving space to people. Just being there was stressed on more than one occasion. Altschul (1984) concluded some years ago that maybe nurses did not have to do anything, they merely had to be there. May and Kelly (1982) however have argued that this makes the job of evaluating a nurse's performance difficult.

Nurses were knowledgeable about a number of approaches to facilitate recovery or change, for example cognitive interventions, but unable to implement these for reasons described earlier. The apparent practice of early discharge, working at a relatively high pace with a rapid turnover of patients were further contributing factors in the nurses' inability to develop therapeutic relationships and interventions.

Nurses were faced in this environment with a wide range of problems that the patients presented themselves with, which, as they indicated, they often felt unskilled to deal with. It may be useful to consider Carr's (1979) point in this context, who has suggested that the psychiatric admission unit may not be a suitable place to care for acutely disturbed patients. Indeed, some nurses felt that the environment did the patients more harm than good.

There were then a variety of reasons why nurses were not in a position to perform an autonomous therapeutic role. Within the setting nurses either adapted to the prevailing ideology and practices, or, as was mentioned, they left.

Dawkins et al (1985), exploring occupational stress among mental health nurses, found that administrative duties and staffing resources concerned nurses most. The findings of this study indicated that staffing levels and the skill mix of staff caused much concern among the respondents. Qualified staff delegated clinical functions to those with limited abilities and knowledge, such as HCA's, who seemed to spend most time with patients, with the most skilled and qualified practitioners engaged in administrative activities, leaving little time for patient contact. Handy (1991) has reported similar findings. The emphasis, reluctantly it seemed, was on managing those members of staff, rather than providing direct patient care. White's (1991) Delphi study suggested that nurses were indeed concerned that a great deal of their time would be taken up with supervising HCA's and that this group would be engaged in most of the patient contact.

Nurses in this study seemed caught between the medically dominated ideology and the interdisciplinary ideology, a point which has been argued by Cox (1986), which left them feeling confused and uncertain. Nurses may favour the interdisciplinary ideology, and stake their claim as independent autonomous practitioners. However, it has been proposed that the traditional hierarchical relationship between doctors and nurses is a difficult one to break (Nolan 1993). One non nurse respondent indeed commented that doctors were in a position to tell nurses what to do.

Nurses were seen to exercise little influence in the multi-disciplinary team, due mainly to their inability to assert themselves in that team and articulate their thoughts and ideas. The hierarchical nursing structure, the dominant medical ideology, but also nurses themselves were given as possible reasons why nurses were so passive in the multi-disciplinary team. Strauss et al (1964) found that nurses were ideologically neutral and adapted to the prevailing ideology. It could be argued that little progress has been made over the last thirty years.

In summary, nurses seemed to have a number of therapeutic skills and qualities, which are considered, in the prescriptive literature, to benefit the recovery of people with mental health problems. However, they were unable to employ those skills and qualities, due to a variety of - on the whole - negative influences, over which they exercised, or felt unable to exercise, little control. This resulted in mainly administrative activities, and care-taking and controlling practices, with little influence in decision making processes.

Some suggestions for training

In recent years, there has been considerable interest, in the concept of the *reflective practitioner* in nursing and psychiatric nursing (Davis and Burnard 1992, Bodley 1992, Alexander 1993, Gray and Pratt 1991). There is a considerable international literature on the topic and much work has been done in Australia and New Zealand on the topic. Usually having its roots in the work of Schon (1983) the argument is usually that psychiatric nurse should learn not only to be effective and skilled carers but also to reflect on what they do as a means of developing their practice. As Alexander (1993) pointed out, such an idea is not one that is readily embraced by *all* nurses. Much work needs to be done to help psychiatric nurses at all levels to develop this reflective and critical practice. In this section, some pointers for teaching reflective and critical skills are described and discussed. It should be borne in mind, at all times, that the concept of reflection is a complex one: exactly how we should define it remains open to question.

As we have acknowledged, the notion of reflective practice is usually linked to the work of Donald Schon (1983) but clearly relates also to educational ideas prior to his writings (Wirth 1979, Freire 1972, Mezirow 1981). Reflection, as an educational tool, has also been advocated by Heron (1973) who described it in terms of 'noticing' or becoming aware of what you are doing, as you are doing it. In the psychiatric nursing field, early papers (Smoyak and Rouslin 1982) describe the *conscious use of the self* as a therapeutic enterprise. The notion involved consciously using certain personal skills in everyday psychiatric nursing practice and thus acting as a reflective practitioner. In other literature, Burnard (1983) and Kilty (1978) have both referred to the idea of learning *through* and *from* experience as part of an experiential learning cycle, which, again involves the practitioner is being aware of his or her own psychological, cognitive and behaviour state. Indeed, reflection may even be described as a particular state of consciousness: consciousness or awareness of events, in the present time and as they happen, with the 'doer' fully aware of his or her intentions as well as his or her actions.

Jarvis (1992) argued that reflective practice was an essential part of nursing as a professional activity. He makes the point that although nursing tends to be a highly structured and ritualised activity, mentors and supervisors can help neophyte psychiatric nurses to develop reflective skills. He also suggests that reflective practice can also help nurses to 'grow' both professionally and personally. One of the distinctive features of reflection, is, perhaps, that no two people's reflections are likely to be the same. This subjective learning process can act as a foil and a contrast to the more formal, lecture-based learning sessions that are now offered in many colleges of nursing.

Developing these themes, this section describes how many of these educational and therapeutic principles can be brought together in educational activities that can be used in a variety of educational settings.

74

Experiential learning

One of the most widely used approaches to encouraging reflection in nurse education is via the use of experiential learning methods. As Weill and McGill (1989) acknowledge, the notion of *experiential learning* can embrace a number of different activities. Sometimes, it is used to indicate that a student has a stock of prior life experience on which to draw. This *must* be the case for all learners: no one comes to a learning encounter as an adult without having built up a large amount of experience from the process of living. In this sense, then, no one comes into nurse education as a 'blank slate'. We can always use and build upon the experience that students bring with them when they start a nursing course.

At other times, and most often in the nursing education litera-ture (Burnard 1991, Kagan 1986), the term *experiential learning* is used as a way of describing certain sorts of group and pairs activities that encourage students to learn by *doing*. The 'doing' is only the first part of the process. What must happen next is that students *reflect* on what they have experienced during a group exercise, a role play or a simulation. It is this process of reflection that helps to reinforce learning. It is also the means by which new learning is added to the existing stock that the student has. Without reflection, it may be argued that the student has merely been through the motions of doing an activity. Reflection can bring personal and idiosyncratic *meaning* to that experience.

Also, this process of reflecting on an educational activity is also a means of learning about the reflective process, itself. In this way, at least *two* things are going on. First, the student is thinking about the group activity or role play. Second, she or he is learning *how* to reflect. Usually, in post-experiential learning activities, the nurse teacher (in the role of facilitator) is empowering those students to spend *time* on reflection. That teacher will encourage the students to consider every aspect of the activity: what it was like to do it, what emotions were experienced, how it links to 'real life nursing' and so on. All of this, slow and considered reflection is part of the process of getting the most out of experiential learning activities. It is also the means by which students can learn how to be quietly and extensively reflective about what they do as nurses. Thus we have a *two level* approach to learning. On that one hand, there is the overt agenda - direct reflection on the experiential learning activity. On the other hand, there is the covert or 'hidden' agenda - the learning about the *process* of reflection. Each time an experiential learning activity is engaged in and is followed by a reflective period, the notion of reflection as a valid and valuable activity is reinforced. This, then, is one method of helping students to become reflective practitioners.

Mentors

Increasingly, in the European literature on nursing education, there is an emphasis on the role of the *mentor* in clinical nursing work (Morle 1990). Although there has been considerable debate as to what, exactly, the role of a mentor might be, most writers are agreed that a clinical mentor should be someone with considerable nursing experience and who can befriend and assist the student nurse in his or her learning process. In the end, it probably doesn't matter so much what such a person is *called*. What matters *very* much is what they *do*. One of the most important tasks for a mentor is to help develop and enhance the reflective abilities of students.

Such reflective work can take a variety of forms. First, the clinically based mentor can set aside time to sit with a student and invite him or her to think about the patients he or she has cared for, how that care was organised and how it might be enhanced in the future. Next, the mentor may encourage the student to link what has been happening with *nursing theory*. Here, we see Freire's (1972) notion of *praxis* (theory in practice) in action. The student is directly linking what he or she *does* in the clinical setting with what others have *written* about nursing and the process of nursing. A number of nursing researchers have identified the 'theory-practice' gap in nursing - the difference between what goes on in the clinical setting and what is written about nursing (see, for example Alexander 1983, Orton 1981). Clinical reflection, of the sort described here, can help to bridge the gap between theory and practice. This is not to deny that there must *always* be something of a gap between the two. If theory always matched practice, then, presumably, some sort of stasis would exist. There would be little to fire and enthuse the practicing nursing and the nursing researcher to develop his or her ideas further. On the other hand, it is essential that the nurse educator does not become so idealistic that he or she looses sight of the real world of nursing. Again, clinical reflective practice can help here.

Diaries

A third method of helping students to develop skills as a reflective practitioner is through the use of a diary (Lyte and Thompson 1990). Such a diary can be used in a variety of ways. First, there is the personal diary that is kept as a 'free-form' document and filled in regularly but with little or not structure to it. With such a diary, the nurse is free to write down his or her thoughts and feelings exactly as they occur. This can, if necessary, later be content analysed (Carney 1982). In this way, it is possible to bring some order to what is, essentially, an unstructured and free flowing document.

Another sort of diary is the *structured* one. Here, a variety of headings is offered to the student and he or she is invited to structure the diary according to those headings. This approach to self-monitoring a psychiatric nursing module of a bachelor's course in nursing has been described elsewhere (Burnard 1988). It seems likely that some degree of structure is likely to be useful in helping students to reflect on their work in a way that is meaningful. Whilst the unstructured approach to diary keeping may be attractive to some students, others find it bewildering. The structure, almost paradoxically, brings the student freedom to express him or herself. The fact that certain 'signposts' are offered as a means of thinking about what has been happening, frees the student up to concentrate on the clinical experience. Suitable headings (which may be adapted according to context) might include the following:

- Clinical skills observed
- Clinical skills performed
- New clinical skills learned
- New references (books, articles, research monographs)
- Personal feelings about the clinical placement
- Things learned this week.

Processing of the diary can take a number of forms. First, it can be used as a reflective instrument, directly in the clinical area. Mentors may encourage students to share their diary entries with each other and to discuss them in small groups.

Alternatively, the mentor can discuss the student's diary with him or her and in private. Again, the reflective approach can be adopted here. Rather than asking direct questions about the student's experience, the mentor uses an approach not unlike the Rogerian, client-centred therapy, advocated by the late Carl Rogers (Rogers 1967). In this approach, the student is encouraged to think about what he or she has written and the mentor merely 'draws out' the student by encouraging him or her to say more and more about what is written. In this way, the experience that is encapsulated in the diary is developed and extrapolated. And, again, the reflective process is being used and reinforced.

Conclusion

These, then, are three ways in which reflection can be developed or even taught to students. All three ways may be described as 'personal'. They encourage the students to involve themselves in the learning process in an active and human way. It is no longer sufficient to see education as being a process of passing on of information. More and more, education is becoming a process of personal as well as intellectual growth. Given the 'caring' nature of nursing (Morrison 1992), this seems to be an important fact. If we really want a workforce that is made up of those who are not only knowledgeable and technically proficient but also sensitive, tactful and caring, then we must encourage students to reflect on their clinical experience and their *personal* experience. The two are, of course, interlinked. You cannot experience a life event without that event affecting *you* in some way. The processes of reflective practice that have been described here are merely ways of making that link explicit.

All of the above, however, still leave open the question of what *exactly* mental health skills might be. For if those skills cannot, precisely, be described, then it is reasonable to suggest that they cannot be *taught*. As always, much teaching in the field of mental health takes its content from *theory* and from *personal practice and personal preference* rather than from research.

6 Conclusion

The aim of this study was to investigate the therapeutic skills that nurses employed in an acute psychiatric admission environment, and factors that influenced the employment of those skills. It was shown that nurses had a range of interpersonal skills, personal qualities and therapeutic approaches on which they could draw, but that various factors prevented them from employing those skills and qualities to their full potential.

The results of the study then seemed to suggest the following:

* Different professional groups held different beliefs about what they do, or should do.

* Nursing in this setting had a predominantly co-ordinating character.

* Nurses had a range of therapeutic skills and qualities, but were hindered in employing these, due to a number of organisational, ideological, managerial and environmental factors.

* Least skilled members of the nursing staff had highest levels of patient contact.

* Nursing care was ad hoc, unstructured and reactive.

*   Nursing care had custodial rather than facilitative characteristics.

*   Nurses were generalist "dogsbodies", assisting other disciplines in the performance of their role.

*   Nurses were valued for their skills in anger management.

Discrepancies between the prescribed and described role of nurse were identified.   The results confirmed the findings of earlier studies undertaken in similar settings (Cormack 1976, 1983; Towell 1975; Carr 1979; Macilwaine 1983; Bunch 1985; Handy 1991).

However, it may be that the vision that the profession holds for mental health nursing in an acute psychiatric environment needs to be adapted.   Towell (1975) found that the occupational label nurse encompassed many different roles, depending on the setting in which the nurse worked.   Connolly (1992) pointed out that there was a need to formulate specific functions for nurses, even if these functions were confined to co-ordinating and integrating the contributions of the various team members. The conclusion may be that nursing in this environment has a predominantly co-ordinating, administrative and managerial character. The implications of Connolly's suggestion, if accepted, seems to be about the role of the nurse in this setting.   However, it is a suggestion that conflicts with present thinking within the mental health nursing profession.

Mauksch (1963) argued that nurses were caught between the cross-roads of accepting a primarily co-ordinating function or a patient centred clinical function. Thirty years later the same argument can be applied here.   Butterworth (1987) claimed that nurses should be recognised as independent agents of therapeutic interventions, but did not make clear where this recognition should come from. He also argued that we must shake off our paternal partnership of medicine and enter into equal partnership with our colleagues in other professions, and that nurses must declare an expertise in interpersonal skills and the therapeutic use of self.

There are many complex, intertwined issues, as has been demonstrated in this study, for nurses to be able to make those decisions independently. Prescribing a role for mental health nurses as autonomous therapeutic agents may be, certainly within the acute psychiatric admission environments, a case of self deception and delusion, which may only lead to further confusion and uncertainty.

The results of this study need to be treated with caution. The researcher adopted a single method, the semi-structured interview. The limitations of this method were discussed earlier. A triangulated approach, as proposed by Denzin (1970), may not only have strengthened the reliability and validity of the results, but may have illuminated the topic under investigation from different angles.

The results were based on data collected almost exclusively in one clinical setting. Descriptive, qualitative studies of this nature intend to explore and highlight certain issues. However, the results seemed to be reliable and valid if compared with earlier studies undertaken in similar settings, and the conclusion can be made that very little has changed during the last twenty-five years in mental health nursing in acute psychiatric admission environments.

A number of recommendations are suggested for the areas of practice, management, education and research.

Nurses and other mental health professionals may find it useful to gain an understanding and seek clarity about each other's role. This may also lead to a clearer identity of the nurse's role. Nurses need to identify what positive contributions they make to the care that patients receive, and convince themselves and others of their value and worth. Nursing management at all levels will need to facilitate and implement change, which will lead to more facilitative practices in patient care. The issue of staffing levels and skill mix also needs to be addressed.

The education of mental health nurses take place in isolation from other professional groups involved in mental health care provision. It has been suggested that this has encouraged isolationist thinking, and has not served patient care very well (Nolan 1993). Interdisciplinary education may be a way of overcoming this isolation between these professional groups, although it is realised that this is opposed by some members of the profession.

Educationalists may also take into account Handy's (1991) point, who argued that the problems of working in a hierarchical institutional context dominated by the medical profession have been ignored in mental health nurse education.

Clarity need to be established as to what student nurses are being prepared for: well informed laymen, with an understanding of some therapeutic approaches, or skilled autonomous practitioners, able to work independently.

It is assumed that the issue of nurses' lack of assertiveness is being addressed through Project 2000, with its aim of producing articulate, assertive, and analytically skilled nurses.

It was interesting to note that nurses were seen as skilled generalists. Nursing in an acute psychiatric admission environment, it seemed, was not considered, by some at least, as a specialist area, in contrast to other areas of mental health nursing, requiring special skills and qualities. Keltner (1985) and Barker (1989) suggested that this may have led to nurses in his setting to feel like second class citizens. A case could be made to recognise this area as a speciality, by creating specific post registration courses.

Finally, a number of research suggestions and ideas are offered, that may shed further light on the issues addressed in this study. A further study into the skills of mental health nurses is warranted, and in particular a study that adopts a variety of approaches, instead of a single method applied in this study. This study, and others in the past, have hinted at possible explanations and reasons why nurses act as they act. It may be useful to gain a better understanding of these various explanations. Porter (1993) suggests that, given the state of flux in mental health nursing, research into the practice and factors influencing this practice is of considerable importance. Hopton (1993) points out that no work on the scale of Barton (1976) has been undertaken in the small psychiatric units attached to District General Hospitals (D.G.H.'s), which now are the most common type of in-patient facility. He suggests that a contemporary analysis of the power relationships between nurses and clients is needed in these environments. The role and function of these units, and its staff, need to be re-examined, which should incorporate an examination of the suitability of these units (D.O.H. 1994a). It is interesting to note that Carr (1979) suggested the same 15 years ago. Not much progress appears to have been made in the intervening years, although alternatives to hospital admission are being explored and examined.

Collaborative approaches, in the form of for example action research generated by practitioners, managers and researchers, may be a useful way, not only to examine some of the areas identified, but to facilitate and bring about change in nursing practice. Closely linked to that is the need to undertake outcome studies, in order to not only identify the contributions of nurses in the care, but also to examine the effectiveness of those contributions.

It is important to view the observations, conclusions and recommendations in the context of the continuing reshaping of mental health services in this country. Future organisational structures may provide mental health nurses with opportunities to practise their skills in a more progressive and dynamic fashion. Nurses themselves however must be actively and proactively involved in creating and implementing innovative services for people with acute mental health problems, in order to realise their therapeutic potential. If they do not, others will do it for them, or do it instead of them.

Appendix 1:
Topics covered during interviews

The frame of reference of the semi-structured interview process centred around the therapeutic skills that nurses employed in an acute psychiatric admission unit. The following areas served as an aide memoire for the researcher during the interviews.

* Understanding of "therapeutic".

* Skills used.

* Unique features.

* Time spent.

* Obstacles.

* Influences.

* Differences.

Appendix 2:
Sample of transcript analysis

This appendix offers part of a transcript, which illustrates the way in which the text was coded.

	Q.	So you have a range of skills available. Are you always in a position to use these skills?
don't use skills	A.	You <u>don't use most of your skills,</u>
constraints		the <u>constraints are very great</u>. Running is a good skill you use here. No, the constraints are
interruptions		great, <u>the interruptions,</u> you're
prioritising need		<u>trying to give somebody time,</u> you <u>cannot let a colleague get beaten</u>

violence common		up, when they shout, you go. That
occurrence		happens on a regular basis.
	Q.	Any others?
time constraint	A.	Time is the factor. In order to come across to somebody, they have to know
developing		that you're willing to give them your
relationships		time, and you got to give them this time beforehand, so they build up this
psychological		psychological safety, so they can
safety		offload and talk to you. All you're able to do is glance around in the
example of time		morning, chat to them over the trolley
constraint		and if there is a catastrophe, spend ten minutes with them. So time is a very important factor, two qualified
staffing constraint		staff per shift, one is in the ward- round all morning, the other doesn't have the time.
	Q.	So you have skills, but you cannot

87

use them?

interest in

cognitive therapy

but not possible

to implement due

time?

staffing?

changing demands?

inability to

provide structure

work

A. That's right. Lots of the time...I
am very <u>interested in the cognitive</u>
<u>therapy and redressing people's</u>
<u>negative thoughts.</u> You try and do it
in passing, but <u>in no way can you get</u>
<u>this across in any meaningful structured</u>
<u>way in this situation.</u> Lots of
times...in the morning, when somebody
is having trouble just getting out of
bed, <u>you can come across with some of</u>
<u>the ideas like cognitive therapy, but</u>
<u>then you're not able to follow it up.</u>
<u>Something else happens</u>, for example
trouble in the canteen. Then the
moment is lost.

Appendix 3:
Annotated interview transcript

This transcript illustrates the way in which the interviews in this study were carried out. The annotations also serve as comment on the process and offer a move towards the type of analysis described in the methodology chapter under the 'alternatives' heading.

RESEARCHER: What therapeutic skills do you employ in this setting, or, what do you do that could be interpreted as therapeutic [1]?

RESPONDENT: As a nurse rather than a manager [2]?

RESEARCHER: Your contributions in relation to nursing care [3].

RESPONDENT: Being a ward manager [4] I try to get involved and use my therapeutic skills, but that's not always possible. You end up [5] co-

---

[1] The researcher asks a multiple question. Also, he attempts to 'broaden' the question with the phrase 'or what do you do that could be *interpreted* as therapeutic'.

[2] The respondent makes a distinction between *nurse* and *manager*. Others may or may not see 'managing' and 'nursing' as part of the same role.

[3] The researcher sticks to a broad definition of nursing.

[4] The respondent makes her own decision about 'which' sort of nurse is under discussion and talks about her work as a manager.

ordinating teams, primary nurses, named nurses and monitoring their input and skills.

RESEARCHER: So you are not in a position to use your therapeutic skills?

RESPONDENT: I do try, input into one-to-one, and groups twice or three times a week[6].

RESEARCHER: So you use certain skills in those situations[7]?

RESPONDENT: On a one-to-one, you use all the skills you've learned during your training and build up such as patience, empathy, try to develop trusting relationships, although that's not always easy, helping people to focus on their problems, giving advice, pointing out alternatives for people which they aren't always able to do for themselves. Try to enable people to be more independent. Education, teaching .[8]..

RESEARCHER: Are these skills different from those that you would use in another setting ? Is there something about the acute setting that differs from other settings ?

RESPONDENT: In acute, sometimes you deal with people who are very disturbed, violent, so you have particular skills, like giving space, although sometimes you have to encroach on people's space, protect other people[9].

---

[5] The respondent 'ends up' doing certain things. This suggests that these may not be part of the prescribed role but are aspects of the job that are 'picked up' as the job evolves. The phrase could also denote a negative value judgment of the fact.

[6] Therapeutic skills appear to be used only on certain occasions and not as part of the general process of being a nurse.

[7] The researcher attempts to clarify this.

[8] The respondent offers a more detailed account of the skills that might be used. They are much more generalized than the previous set that were offered.

[9] The respondent introduces the notion of 'giving space' but does not specify what this might be.

RESEARCHER: You've referred to counselling skills, skills dealing with potentially aggressive behaviours, disturbed behaviours, you also mentioned something about groups[10] ?

RESPONDENT: There is a patient group every morning, groups at weekends, although this isn't a set pattern, but we do try to have groups at weekends, time permitting. The inpatient morning group is a very difficult group to run, it's between the two wards, it can sometimes be a very large and often quite disturbed group. We try to select patients you feel are appropriate to benefit from the group[11].

RESEARCHER: Do nurses run these groups ?

RESPONDENT: Mainly by nurses, sometimes they are co-facilitated by a psychologist or by an O.T., but nurses keep the group going. It can be difficult, because you're not there everyday, due to the nature of the shift system. Sometimes issues carry over, and if you are not aware, it can be difficult[12].

RESEARCHER: Does working in a setting like this require special preparation ? What is special about this work [13]?

RESPONDENT: You do need special skills. Most of us have gone through the same RMN curriculum, not everybody is up to it[14]. Personal

---

[10] The researcher picks, particularly, on *counselling* and *groups*.

[11] The respondent talks about groups but not about counselling.

[12] The respondent acknowledges that it is not always nurses who run these groups.

[13] The respondent asks about 'special preparation'. There is a suggestion, here, that such preparation may or may not be above and beyond basic training as a nurse.

[14] Respondent gives an ambiguous reply. She suggests that although 'most of us have gone through the same RMN curriculum (Registered Mental Nurse) - 'not everybody is up to it'. She suggests, that *personal skills* are required. Is she hinting that some people have *personal qualities* that others do not?

skills, you need to be able to work under pressure a lot of the time. Not everybody can work under that pressure and stress[15].

RESEARCHER: Personal skills or qualities ? What personal qualities do you have ?

RESPONDENT: Trying to remain calm, model a calm approach, patients pick up straight away if you cannot handle situations. So modelling a calm approach, even if you don't feel calm.

RESEARCHER: Being a role model. Are there though situations where you think you've come to the end of your tether, "I have no more skills available, I need other health care professionals to help me out" ? Can you give any examples ?[16]

RESPONDENT: I've never worked in an eating disorder unit, or have much experience, so in that situation I'm quite happy to call upon the experts[17]. We do this at the moment. Or adolescents, we have touched upon it in training, but unless you've worked in such a unit, they need specialised skills.

RESEARCHER: But nursing here is specialised all the same. Or isn't it?

RESPONDENT: That's difficult, because you're the only facility in the area, you tend to take whatever comes through the door[18]. Only after that can you decide whether a person needs more specialised skills.

---

[15] Respondent acknowledges the stressful nature of the work. She also acknowledges that trained staff should be *role models* for students.

[16] Researcher changes tack a little and asks for examples of when the researcher has 'used up' all her skills.

[17] Respondent acknowledges an example of her limitations - working with those who have eating disorders and working with adolescents. She also alludes to the idea that you need *experience of working in the field* in order to gain the skills in these fields.

[18] Respondent refers to 'taking whatever comes through the door' and seems to depersonalize the patient group for a moment. She suggests, also, that an assessment

RESEARCHER: Are you a master or jack of all trades in that case ?

RESPONDENT: You tend to be a jack of all trades, but not necessarily master of none. You can be a master of some of them e.g. people with psychosis[19]. I tend to think I'm better skilled with those people rather than people with anxiety, but because we cover the whole of the area, we cannot be that preferential. What we try to do after admission is look at what special skills, experience members of staff have to decide on a primary nurse for patients e.g. somebody with experience in griefwork, then you try to allocate that to a nurse with those skills. But it isn't always possible.

RESEARCHER: Are there skills you could benefit from developing that you do not have at the moment ?

RESPONDENT: Take myself, although we covered a fair deal of griefwork, I felt I was lacking in those skills, so I've decided to do a course looking at that[20].

RESEARCHER: Any other skills ? Or is there such a variety that it would be impossible to cover ?

RESPONDENT: That's right, it's such a broad area, that's the problem, given that we're a hospital that covers a catchment area, you cannot pick or choose the problems that your clients come in with. We tend to take a broad spectrum, apart from the age limit, although even then we have to admit sometimes, because of shortage of beds. That can be problematic, because your skills of working with elderly people can be a bit rusty,

---

phase follows in which it is determined whether or people need 'more specialized skills'.

[19] A specific field of expertise is acknowledged - that of working with psychotic people. Respondent acknowledges more skill in this field than in certain others. She talks of allocating staff to suit patients who need specific skills.

[20] Respondent identifies a need for further training in grief work.

when you're dealing with acutely ill people al the time. So we take all and sundry, you cannot refuse[21].

RESEARCHER: Apart from being a ward manager, which may prevent you from using your skills, what other factors are there[22] ?

RESPONDENT: Staffing levels spring to mind, and administrative work, sometimes you know somebody is on the ward in tears, who needs to speak to someone, and you've got a wardround to go to, write an account of how 14 patients spent the morning, and that can be difficult, dividing your time. H.C.A.'s (health care assistants) are on the ward, but they're not particularly trained. They may be skilled, but that's not brought out, they haven't got the correct training. To give time to all patients isn't always possible, which leads to frustrations. As a ward manager you can sit in the office, doing an off-duty, and then you have people who need time[23].

RESEARCHER: How much time then do nurses spend in therapeutic interactions with their clients [24]?

RESPONDENT: It's difficult, but on average a primary nurse spends about 1/3 of the shift in direct patient contact[25].

RESEARCHER: Is that a fair balance ?

---

[21] Reference is made, again, to 'not refusing' people who come through the door. There is a suggestion, along with the references to stress, that the respondent is finding the job difficult and that it may not be living up to expectations.

[22] Researcher asks a question that invites 'problems' from the researcher.

[23] The respondent refers to all of the 'problems' that stop her from functioning probably.

[24] The researcher changes tack and asks about time spent in therapeutic interactions.

[25] The respondent offers a fairly specific estimate of time allocated to 'direct patient contact' - although this is not the same thing, perhaps, as being 'in therapeutic interactions'.

RESPONDENT: No, but what is ? 2/3 ? It's difficult to say, you have to take time out to plan, to document[26].

RESEARCHER: What are the unique contributions of nurses within the multi-disciplinary team framework [27]?

RESPONDENT: As a nurse your contribution...the MDT get together to discuss a group of patients e.g. in a wardround setting or get discussed each morning. What seems to be happening often that grieves me - I'm not sure whether I should be saying this - is that nurses tend more and more to be information givers i.e. parrots just sitting there, just giving out information. Other people then take away this info and do something with it. This seems to be happening more and more and a nurse's opinion isn't even asked for, unless you push for it[28].

RESEARCHER: Does it have to be asked for ?

RESPONDENT: Unfortunately, although we talk about a MDT, by the very name "wardround" is it still very much consultant dominated. Sometimes it takes a very assertive nurse to get their voice heard[29].

RESEARCHER: What has that got to do with ? Power [30]?

RESPONDENT: Power, old fashioned ideas. The nurses' contributions, the O.T.'s contributions, the S.W's contributions instead of a free forum

---

[26] There is a suggestion that the other two thirds of the time might be taken up with administrative work.

[27] The researcher attempts to pin down the 'uniqueness' of the nurse's role.

[28] The response seems less than specific and suggests that the nurse is a fairly minor player in the ward round. Also, she suggests that the nurse is an 'information giver' to other multidisciplinary team members.

[29] A opinion about the nature of the wardround is expressed and it is acknowledged that it is very much dominated by the consultant. The researcher suggests that nurses need to be more assertive.

[30] The researcher 'leads', here, by suggesting that 'power' might be the 'cause' of the consultant domination of the wardround.

where everyone can speak freely. That's very much a negative side. On a positive side I would like to say that nurses are there as patients' advocates, represent patients, with their consent, discussions from one-to-one counselling, and get different perspectives and ideas, that's how I try to work on it, on a more positive note. Sharing ideas.[31]

RESEARCHER: Has it something to do then with a nurse's experience e.g. years qualified, where they qualified ?

RESPONDENT: Sometimes yes, but also personalities[32].

RESEARCHER: It sounds from what you say that nurses collect data and others do something with it. What are nurses doing with the data [33]?

RESPONDENT: Sometimes we do something with it... but at times it feels as if we're talking machines; the worrying thing is that it is a one way process, you don't get any feedback[34].

RESEARCHER: How different then are your skills in relation to other professionals ?What is unique about nursing, where does it conflict or overlap ? What do you offer that's unique [35]?

RESPONDENT: There are overlapping areas, that's why there is often conflict in MDT forums[36].

---

[31] The respondent offers a much broader range of skills, here: patients' advocacy, patients' representation, discussion, counselling and sharing ideas.

[32] Again, the idea of the nurse's *personality* is raised. Is this as important or even *more* important than particular skills?

[33] The researcher introduces the idea of 'data collection', which may or may not be understood by the respondent.

[34] The respondent bemoans the lack of 'feedback' but it is not clear from whom feedback might be forthcoming.

[35] The researcher tries, again, to get the respondent to be specific about the unique nature of the skills that a nurse can offer. This begs the question as to whether or not nurses' skills *are* unique.

RESEARCHER: Where is the overlap ?

RESPONDENT: E.g. if there's a need to do marital work with a patient and her husband. Consultant is present, junior doctor is present, but the primary nurse is not available, so the O.T. stepped in. The O.T. obviously thought she had those skills. The same with relaxation techniques, nurses have them, but primarily it tends to be an O.T., happening in an O.T. department, but it is something we can do. There are so many overlapping areas.

RESEARCHER: Just with O.T.'s ?

RESPONDENT: Also with Social Work (S.W.), not so much with psychologists. They tend to keep very much to themselves. There isn't much sharing of ideas. Probably we work closer with O.T.'s that there is so much overlap.

RESEARCHER: More conflict than complementary ?

RESPONDENT: Again it sometimes comes down to personalities. It can complement well e.g. someone is admitted and as part of assessment and planning we try to do that as a joint nurse and O.T. venture. Sit down together with the client and discuss the package of care, identify where the nurse and where the O.T. fit in without too much overlap[37].

RESEARCHER: O.T.'s seem to offer more structure, their skills seem more visible than the skills of nurses, which begs the question: what do nurses do here, is it possible to gain a picture, is there a structure to their work ? Or is it crisis management, working ad hoc ?

RESPONDENT: No, it's very much planned e.g. this afternoon there is an O.T. outing, a social activity. A nurse has to go as well, an O.T. cannot take responsibility to take patients out. But then again, is the nurse there as

---

[36] The respondent notes that skills are *overlapping* with other team members.

[37] After discussing areas of skill overlap, the respondent refers, again, to 'personalities'. This is a recurrent theme in this interview.

a custodian, a guardian. A lot of the work is planned, but a lot of it is also crisis management.

RESEARCHER: Nurses apparently are therapeutic agents. Does nursing make a difference ? How do you know that what you've done is your contribution ?

RESPONDENT: A lot of it depends on how many staff you have on duty and how busy the environment is, how many disturbed people you have; you can do some extremely good work with a disturbed person, studying behaviour, looking at the antecedents, seeing how we can interact. It's a standing joke that when a patient becomes disturbed in O.T., they call for a nurse. Why is that ? Because a nurse can come down to give an injection, or because she can utilise her skills, modelling a calm approach[38].

RESEARCHER: So you are a therapeutic agent, not a custodian ?

RESPONDENT: I'd like to think I am, but that is probably telling fibs. But there are overlapping areas. On the whole you can think you're a therapeutic agent, but there are times, where you have to step in, to be a custodian e.g. secluding someone to protect others or individual himself, although you can also say you're a therapeutic agent by doing that. If you're not a custodian, then you're not managing the environment.

RESEARCHER: Anything you would like to add ?

RESPONDENT: Some things need further thinking e.g. issues regarding us and O.T.'s. There are things like handover, what interactions you've had with people over the weekend, then the O.T. goes to the wardround and says such and such was this and this, and you think, she only knows this because I told her, not because of her personal interaction. You think, that was my hard work, my hours spent to build and get some trust and then they (O.T.) take the credit, which can be very frustrating. You try to be

---

[38] An answer to a question about 'therapeutic skills' is met with an answer about the tension between being therapeutic and serving a custodial role. The custodial role had not been referred to, before, in the interview.

rational about it, thinking we're here for the patient and as long as the information is relayed, does it matter, but my it is hard work and skills that I've used. You don't want praise, but it is frustrating[39].

RESEARCHER: Do nurses give too many skills away ?

RESPONDENT: The extent of training of RMN isn't that long, but O.T.'s - I don't want to pick on them - spent about six months in psychiatry out of their three years. I could not be expected to work as a nurse with that length of training[40].

RESEARCHER: Who is given them away ?

RESPONDENT: We are, it seems[41].

RESEARCHER: Earlier you mentioned your managerial, and administrative duties, could that be done by someone else ?

RESPONDENT: I think so, yes, that's why it's so frustrating. I trained to be a nurse, I enjoy nursing in an acute setting; doing silly things like answering telephones, somebody else could do that, take messages. I was seeing somebody the other day whom I knew had been upset during the morning, who needed to speak to somebody; I'd been speaking to her for about 20 minutes, and was interrupted by a ward clerk: Senior Nurse Manager wants to see you". "Cannot, I'm busy now". "It's urgent". Drop all tools, leave patient with all her feelings.

RESEARCHER: Administration seems valued higher by senior management than your clinical expertise. Failing your administrative duties is spotted easier and seen as more important than failing your clinical duties and responsibilities.

---

[39] This answer suggests some tension between the different disciplines and a sense that the respondent feels undervalued in her role.

[40] The respondent notes a discrepancy between the length of a psychiatric nurses' training and that of an occupational therapist.

[41] The respondent feels that nurses 'give away' their skills.

RESPONDENT: I couldn't agree more, but it happens. Establishment figures have higher priority than talking to a distressed client. You make arrangements to see clients, you make sure the ward is covered, but you still get interrupted. That's the frustration of a lot of nurses[42].

RESEARCHER: There seems to be a frightening development with HCA's, as you described earlier ?

RESPONDENT: Being frank about it, we've got far too many, too many untrained HCA's, just out of school. I've got 4 here who haven't even been to the basic course. 7 or 8 here is far too many, compared to your ratio of 2 qualified members and 3 HCA's on a shift. Qualified staff have the skills[43].

RESEARCHER: Are HCA's replacing qualified staff and students ?

RESPONDENT: Yes, in some ways, skillmix is changing, but they are so inadequately and ill prepared for their role, standards are dropping[44].

RESEARCHER: Is that noticeable ?

RESPONDENT: We don't move people forward as quickly as we could, that's the main thing[45].

RESEARCHER: But you need to make the case: "these HCA's have had a negative effect on patient care", but you must be able to prove that[46].

---

[42] After a discussion about the administrative work that nurses have to do, the question that still remains, unanswered, is 'what would nurses do if they did not do administrative work?'

[43] The respondent notes that 'qualified nurses "have the skills"' and suggest that untrained helpers do not.

[44] Skills are noted to be dropping and this is related to a change in the 'skill mix'.

[45] An indicator of 'standards dropping' is the inability of the team to 'move people forward'. It is not clear what this means.

[46] The researcher appears to be offering advice about how to change the situation.

RESPONDENT: Qualified staff are the parrots in the office[47], planning care, handovers to others. HCA's are on the wards, hardly knowing how to deal with situations/problems, it's not fair on them, not fair on qualified staff; you end up overburdened, frustrated, overworked, often that frustration is vented on to them (HCA's), thinking: "why don't you think".

---

[47] Nurses are described as 'the parrots of the office'.

References

Abrahams, P. (1984) Evaluating Soft Findings : Some Problems of Measuring Informal Care, Research, *Policy and Planning*, 2, 2, 1-8.

Adams, A. (1991) Paradigms in psychiatric nursing, *Nursing, 4, 35, 9-11.*

Alexander, M. E. (1983) *Learning to Nurse: Integrating Theory and Practice*, Churchill Livingstone, Edinburgh.

Alexander, M.E. (1993) Promoting Analytical and Critical Thinking in Nursing: With Particular Emphasis on the Post-Registration Education of Qualified Nurses and Midwifes, *Asian Journal of Nursing Studies*, Inaugural Issue.

Allport, G. (1942) *The use of personal documents in psychological science*, Social Science Research Council, New York.

Altschul, A. (1972) *Patient-nurse interactions: a study of interaction patterns in acute psychiatric wards*, Churchill Livingstone, Edinburgh.

Altschul, A. (1984) Does good practice need good principles? *Nursing Times, July 18, 49-51.*

American Nurses' Association (1980) *Nursing: a policy statement,* Kansas City, Missouri.

Argyris, C. and Schon, D. (1976) *Theory into practice: increasing professional effectiveness,* Jossey Bass, San Francisco.

Arthur, D., Dowling, J. and Sharkey, R. (1992) *Mental health nursing: strategies for working with the difficult client,* Harcourt Brace Javanovich, Sydney.

Ashworth, P.D., Giorgi, A. and de Koning, A.J.J. (eds) (1986) Qualitative Research in Psychology, *Proceedings of the International Association for Qualitative Research,* Duquesne University Press, Pittsburgh, PA.

Audit Commission (1994) *Finding a place: a review of mental health services for adults,* HMSO, London.

Bamber, M. (1988) Quitting, *Nursing Times,* 84,22,33-34.

Barber, P. (1986) The psychiatric nurse's failure therapeutically to nurture, *Nursing Practice, 1, 138-141.*

Barker, P. (1989) Bridging the gap, *Nursing Standard, 3, 20, 22-24.*

Barker, P. (1990) The conceptual basis of mental health nursing, *Nurse Education Today, 10, 339-348.*

Barker, P. (1994) A partnership for change, *Nursing Times,* 90,20,62.

Barton, R. (1976) *Institutional neurosis,* Wright, London.

Bell, C. and Newby, H. (eds) (1977) *Doing Sociological Research,* Allen and Unwin, London.

Berg, B. (1989) *Qualitative research methods for the social sciences,* Allyn and Bacon, New York.

Berg, B.L. (1989) *Qualitative Research Methods for the Social Sciences* : Allyn and Bacon, New York.

Berne, E. (1964) *Games people play,* Grove Press, New York.

Bodley, D.E. (1992) Clinical Supervision in Psychiatric Nursing: Using the Process Record, *Nurse Education Today,* 12, 148-155.

Brenner, M. (1985) Intensive interviewing. In: M. Brenner, J. Brown, and D. Canter (eds) *The research interview: uses and approaches,* Academic Press, London.

Brenner, M., Brown, J. and Canter, D. (eds) (1985) *The research interview: uses and approaches,* Academic Press, London.

Brooking, J. (1985) Advanced psychiatric nursing education in Britain, *Journal of Advanced Nursing, 10, 455-468.*

Brooking, J. (ed) (1986) *Psychiatric nursing research,* J. Wiley and Sons, Chichester.

Brooking, J., Ritter, S. and Thomas, B. (eds) (1992) *A textbook of psychiatric and mental health nursing,* Churchill Livingstone, Edinburgh.

Brown, D. and Pedder, J. (1991) *Introduction to psychotherapy: an outline of psychodynamic principles and practice,* Tavistock/Routledge, London.

Brown, D., Carson, J., Fagin, L., Bartlett, H. and Leary, J. (1994) Coping with caring, *Nursing Times,* 90,45,53-55.

Bryman, A. (1988) *Quantity and Quality in Social Research,* Unwin Hyman, London.

Bunch, E. (1985) Therapeutic communication: is it possible for psychiatric nurses to engage in this on an acute psychiatric ward? In: A. Altschul (ed) *Psychiatric Nursing,* Churchill Livingstone, Edinburgh.

Burgess, R. (1984) *In the field: an introduction to field research,* Unwin Hyman, London.

Burnard, P. (1988) The Journal as an Assessment and Evaluation Tool in Nurse Education, *Nurse Education Today*, 8, 105-107.

Burnard, P. (1989) Fads and fashions, *Nursing Times, 85, 8, 69-71, Feb 22.*

Burnard, P. (1991) A method of analysing interview transcripts in qualitative research, *Nurse Education Today, 11, 461-466.*

Burnard, P. (1991) *Experiential Learning in Action,* Avebury, Aldershot.

Burnard, P. and Morrison, P. (1990) *Nursing research in action: developing basic skills,* MacMillan, London.

Butterworth, A. (1987) Psychiatric nursing: fumbling in a vacuum, or grasping at opportunity, *Mental Health Nursing, 1, 7, Sept.*

Butterworth, A. (1991) Generating research in mental health nursing, *International Journal of Nursing Studies, 28, 3, 237-246.*

Carney, J. (1982) *Content Analysis,* Harper and Row, London.

Carr, P. (1979) *To describe the role of the psychiatric nurse in a psychiatric unit which is situated in a district general hospital complex,* Ph.D. Thesis, University of Manchester.

Chenitz, W. C. and Swanson, J. M. (1986) *From Practice to Grounded Theory: Qualitative Research in Nursing,* Addison Wesley, Menlo Park, California.

Cicourel, A. (1964) *Method and measurement in sociology,* The Free Press, New York.

Clarke, L. (1988) Ideology, tradition and choice: questions psychiatric nurses ask themselves, *Senior Nurse, 8, 11, 11-13.*

Cohen, L. and Manion, L. (1985) *Research methods in education,* (2nd Ed), Croom Helm, London.

Connolly, M. (1992) Issues and developments in psychiatric nursing: history. In: J. Brooking, S. Ritter, and B. Thomas (eds) *A textbook of psychiatric and mental health nursing,* Churchill Livingstone, Edinburgh. Cormack, D. (1976) *Psychiatric nursing observed,* Royal College of Nursing, London.

Cormack, D. (1983) *Psychiatric nursing described,* Churchill Livingstone, Edinburgh.

Cormack, D.F.S. (1984) *The Research Process in Nursing,* Blackwell, Oxford.

Corwin, R. (1961) Role conception and career aspiration: a study of identity in nursing, *Sociological Quarterly, 2, 69-86.*

Cox, B. (1990) Nurse and empathy: psychiatric nursing today, *The Canadian Journal of Nursing Research, 22, 3, 19-22.*

Crabtree, B. and Miller, W. (ed) (1992) *Doing qualitative research,* Sage, California.

Davis, B. (1981) Trends in psychiatric nursing research, *Nursing Times, June 25, 73-76, Occasional Paper.*

Davis, B. (1986) A review of recent research in psychiatric nursing. In: J. Brooking (ed) *Psychiatric nursing research,* J. Wiley and Sons, Chichester.

Davis, B. (1990) Research and psychiatric nursing. In: W. Reynolds and D. Cormack (eds) *Psychiatric and mental health nursing: theory and practice,* Chapman and Hall, London.

Davis, B.D. and Burnard, P. (1992) Academic Levels in Nursing, *Journal of Advanced Nursing*, 17, 1395-1400.

Dawkins, J., Depp, F. and Selzer, N. (1985) Occupational stress in a public mental health hospital, *Journal of Psychosocial Nursing and Mental Health Services, 23, 8-15.*
Dean, C. and Gadd, E. (1990) Home treatment for acute psychiatric illness, *British Medical Journal,* 301,6759,1021-1023.

Denzin, N. (1970) *The research act,* Aldine, Chicago.
Department of Health (1994a) *Working in partnership: a collaborative approach to care,* HMSO, London.

Department of Health (1994b) *Mental health in London: priorities for action. A Mental Health Task Report,* D.O.H., London.

Emerson, R. (ed) (1983) *Contemporary field research,* Little Brown, Boston.

Emrich, K. (1989) Helping or hurting: interacting in the therapeutic milieu, *Journal of Psychosocial Nursing, 27, 12, 26-29.*

English National Board (1982) *Syllabus of training - Professional Register - Part 3 (Registered Mental Nurse),* English National Board, London.

Farrington, A. (1992) Mental health nursing: now you see it, now you don't, *British Journal of Nursing, 1, 6, 272.*

Faugier, J. (1994) Thin on the ground, *Nursing Times,* 90,20,64-65.

Ferguson, K. (1992) *Position Paper on in-patient psychiatric nursing,* D.O.H., London.

Field, P.A. and Morse, J. M (1985) *Nursing Research: The Application of Qualitative Approaches*, Croom Helm, London.

Fink, A. and Kosekoff, J. (1985) *How to do Surveys*, Sage, Beverly Hills, California.

Footwhyte, F. (1982) Interviewing in field research. In: R. Burgess (ed) *Field research: a sourcebook and field manual*, Allen Unwin, London.

Freire, P. (1972) *Pedagogy of the Oppressed*, Penguin, Harmond-sworth.

Gallop, R., Lancee, W. and Garfinkel, P. (1990) The expressed empathy of psychiatric nursing staff, *The Canadian Journal of Nursing Research*, *22, 3, 7-18*.

Glaser, B. and Strauss, A.L.. (1967) *The Discovery of Grounded Theory*, Aldine, New York.

Gray, P. and Pratt, T. (1993) *Towards a Discipline of Nursing*, Churchill Livingstone, Edinburgh.

Guba, E. and Lincoln, Y. (1981) *Effective evaluation*, Jossey Bass, San Francisco.

Handy, J. (1991) The social context of occupational stress in a caring profession, *Social Science Medicine, 32, 7, 819-830*.

Heron, J. (1973) *Experiential Training Techniques*, University of Surrey, Guildford.

Heron, J. (1990) *Helping the client: a creative practical guide*, Sage, London.

Hockey, L. (1991) Foreword. In: R. McMahon and A. Pearson (eds) *Nursing as Therapy*, Chapman and Hall, London.

Hopton, J. (1993) The contradictions of mental health nursing, *Nursing Standard*, 8,11,37-39.

Isles, J. (1986) An identity crisis perpetuated, *Nursing Times, June 18, 28-32*.

Jarvis, P. (1992) Reflective Practice and Nursing, *Nurse Education Today*, 12, 174-181.

John, A. (1961) *A study of the psychiatric nurse*, E and S Livingstone, Edinburgh.

Joint Committee of Mental Health Nursing Organisations (1986) *The role of the psychiatric nurse*, Psychiatric Nursing Association, Littlemore, Oxford.

Kagan, C. Evans, J. and Kay, B. (1986) (eds) *A Manual of Interpersonal Skills: An Experiential Approach*, Harper and Row, London.

Keltner, N. (1985) Psychotherapeutic management: a model for nursing practice, *Perspectives in Psychiatric Care, 23, 4, 125-130.*

Kerr, N. (1990) Ego competency: a framework for formulating the nursing care plan, *Perspectives in Psychiatric Care, 26, 4, 30-35.*

Kilty, J. 1978 Self and Peer Assessment: Human Potential Research Project, University of Surrey, Guidford.

Kirk, J.A. and Miller, M.L. (1986) *Reliability and Validity and Qualitative Methods*, Sage, Beverly Hills, California.

Knapp, M.,Beecham, J., Koutsogeorgopoulou, V., Hallam, A., Fenyo, A., Marks, I., Audini, B. and Muijen, M. (1994) Service use and costs of home-based versus hospital-based care for people with serious mental illness, *The British Journal of Psychiatry*, 165,195-204.

Krippendorf, K. (1980) *Content Analysis: an Introduction to its Methodology*, Sage, Beverly Hills, California.

Kvale, S. (1983) The qualitative research interview: a phenomenological and hermeneutical mode of understanding. *Journal of Phenomenological Psychology*, 14, 2, 171-196.

Lacey, D. (1993) Discovering theory from psychiatric nursing practice, *British Journal of Nursing*, 2,15,763-766.

Leys, S. (1986) *The Burning Forest, Essays on Chinese Culture and Politics*, Holt, Rinehart and Winston, New York.

Lutzen, K. (1990) Moral sensing and ideological conflict: aspects of the therapeutic relationship in psychiatric nursing, *Scandinavian Journal of Caring Sciences, 4, 2, 69-76.*

Lyotard, J-F. (1983) *Answering the Question: What is Postmodernism?* In I. Hassan and S. Hassan (eds) *Innovation/renovation*, University of Wisconsin Press, Madison, Wisconsin.

Lyte, V.J. and Thompson, I.G. (1990) The Diary as a Formative Teaching and Learning Aid, *Nurse Education Today*, 10, 228-232.

Macilwaine, H. (1983) The communication patterns of female neurotic patients with nursing staff in psychiatric units. In: J. Wilson-Barnett (ed) *Nursing research: ten studies in patient care*, J. Wiley and Sons, Chichester.

Man Cheung Chung and Nolan, P. (1994) The influence of positivistic thought on nineteenth century asylum nursing, *Journal of Advanced Nursing*, 19,226-232.

Marks, I. and Scott, R. (1990) *Mental health care delivery: innovations, impediments and implementation*, Cambridge University Press, Cambridge.

Marks, I., Connolly, J., Muijen, M., Audini, B., McNamee, G. and Lawrence, R. (1994) Home-based versus hospital-based care for people with serious mental illness, *The British Journal of Psychiatry*, 165,179-195.

Maslach, C. and Jackson, S. (1986) *Maslach Burnout Inventory*, Consulting Psychologists Press, California.

Mauksch, H. (1963) Becoming a nurse: a selective view, *Annals of the American Academy of Political and Social Science, 346, 88-98.*

May, D. and Kelly, M. (1982) Chancers, pests and poor wee souls: problems of legitimation in psychiatric nursing, *Sociology of Health and Illness, 4, 3, 279-301.*

McMahon, R. and Pearson, A. (eds) (1991) *Nursing as therapy,* Chapman and Hall, London.

Measor, L. (1985) Interviewing: a strategy in qualitative research. In: R. Burgess (ed) *Strategies in educational research: qualitative methods,* Falmer Press, London.

Mezirow, J. (1981) A Critical Theory of Adult Learning and Education, *Adult Education,* 32, 1, 3-24.

Miles, M. and Huberman, M. (1984) *Qualitative data analysis: a data source book,* Sage, London.

Miles, M. B. and Huberman, A. M. (1994) *Qualitative Data Analysis,* 2nd Edition, Sage, Thousands Oak, California.

Miles, M.B. (1979) Qualitative data as an attractive nuisance. The problem of analysis. *Administrative Science Quaterly,* 24, 590-601.

Ministry of Health (1968) *Psychiatric nursing: today and tomorrow,* HMSO, London.

Morle, K.M. F. (1990) Mentorship - is it a case of the emperors new clothes or a rose by any other name. *Nurse Education Today,* 10, 66-69.

Morrison, P. (1992) *Professional Caring in Practice,* Avebury, Aldershot.

Morse, J. (ed) (1991) *Qualitative nursing research: a contemporary dialogue,* Sage, California.

Mostyn, B. (1985) The content analysis of qualitative research data: a dynamic approach. In: M. Brenner, J. Brown and D. Canter (eds) *The research interview: uses and approaches,* Academic Press, London.

Munhall, P.L. and Oiler, C.J. (eds) (1986*) Nursing Research: a Qualitative Perspective,* Appleton-Century-Crofts, Newalk, Connecticut.
Nolan, P. (1993) *A history of mental health nursing,* Chapman and Hall, London.

Office of Health Economics (1989) *Mental health in the 1990's: from custody to care,* Office of Health Economics, London.

Oiler, C. (1982) The Phenomenological Approach in Nursing Research, *Nursing Research,* 31, 178-181.

Oppenheim, A. (1955) *The function and training of mental nurses,* Chapman and Hall, London.

Oppenheim, A. (1992) *Questionnaire design, interviewing and attitude measurement,* (new ed) Pinter, London.

Peplau, H. (1952) *Interpersonal relations in nursing,* Putnam, New York.

Peplau, H. (1987) Tomorrow's world, *Nursing Times, Jan 7, 29-31.*

Polanyi, M. (1967) *The tacit dimension,* Doubleday, New York.

Porter, S. (1993) The determinants of psychiatric nursing practice: a comparison of sociological perspectives, *Journal of Advanced Nursing,* 18,1559-1566.

Reed, P. (1987) Constructing a conceptual framework for psychosocial nursing, *Journal of Psychosocial Nursing, 25, 2, 24-28.*

Reynolds, W. and Cormack, D. (1990) *Psychiatric and mental health nursing: theory and practice,* Chapman and Hall, London.

Riley, J. (1990) *Getting the most from your data: a handbook of practical ideas on how to analyse qualitative data,* Technical and Educational Services Ltd, Bristol.

Rogers, C. (1951) *Client-centred therapy,* Constable, London.

Rogers, C.R. (1967) *On Becoming a Person,* Constable, London.
Rolfe, G. (1990) The assessment of therapeutic attitudes in the psychiatric setting, *Journal of Advanced Nursing, 15, 564-570.*

Royal College of Psychiatrists (1994) *Monitoring inner London mental illness services,* Royal College of Psychiatrists, London.

Sandelowski, M. (1986) The problem of rigour in qualitative research, *Advanced Nursing Science, 8, 3, 27-37.*

Schon, D. (1983) *The Reflective Practitioner,* Basic Books, New York.

Silverman, D. (1985) *Qualitative Research Methodology in Sociology,* Gower, Aldershot.

Sloboda, J. (1993) *What is skill and how is it acquired ?* In: Thorpe, M., Edwards, R. and Hanson, A. (eds): *Culture and processes of adult learning,* Routledge, London.

Smith, L. (1988) Far to go? *Nursing Times, 84, 27, 30-32.*

Smith, N.L. (1992) Towards the Justification of Claims in Evaluation Research, *Evaluation and Program Planning, 10, 209-314.*

Smoyak, A.S. and Rouslin, S. (1982) *A Collection of Classics in Psychiatric Nursing Literature,* Slack, Thorofare, New Jersey.

Sommer, B. and Sommer, R. (1991) *A practical guide to behavioural research: tools and techniques,* (3rd ed), Oxford University Press, Oxford.

Strauss, A., Schatzman, L. and Bucher, R. (1964) *Psychiatric ideologies and institutions,* Free Press, Glencoe, New Jersey.

Strauss, A., Schatzman, L., Ehrlich, D., Bucher, R. and Sabshin, M. (1981) *Psychiatric ideologies and institutions,* 2nd ed., Transaction, New Brunswick, New Jersey.

Strauss, A.L. (1987) *Qualitative Data Analysis for Social Scientists,* Cambridge University Press, Cambridge.

Strupp, H. (1986) The nonspecific hypothesis of therapeutic effectiveness: a current assessment, *American Journal of Orthopsychiatry, 56, 4, 513-519.*

Taylor, S. and Bogdan, R. (1984) *Introduction to qualitative research methods: the search for meanings,* (2nd ed), J. Wiley and Sons, New York.

Tesch, R. (1990) *Qualitative research: analysis types and software tools,* Falmer Press, New York.

Thomas, B. (1992) Advances in the clinical practice of psychiatric nursing, *British Journal of Nursing, 1, 6, 292-295.*

Towell, D. (1975) *Understanding psychiatric nursing,* Royal College of Nursing, London.

Turner-Crowson, J. (1993) *Reshaping mental health services: implications for Britain of U.S. experience,* King's Fund Institute, London.

van Manen, M. (1977) Linking ways of knowing with ways of being practical, *Curriculum Inquiry,* 6, 3, 205-228

Vousden, M. (1986) Agents of change, or care-givers? *Nursing Times, June 25, 51-52.*

Walker, R. (1983) Three good reasons for not doing case studies in curriculum research, *Journal of Curriculum Studies, 15, 2, 155-165.*

Ward, M. (1993) Culture shock, *Nursing Times,* 89,21,38-40.

Wardle, M and Mandle, C. (1989) Conceptual models used in nursing practice, *Western Journal of Nursing Research, 11, 1, 108-114.*

Weill, S. W. and McGill, I. (eds) *Making Sense of Experiential Learning,* Open University Press, Milton Keynes.

Weir, R. (1992) An experimental course of lectures on moral treatment for mentally ill people, *Journal of Advanced Nursing,* 17,390-395.

White, E. (1991) *The future of psychiatric nursing by the year 2000: a Delphi study,* Department of Nursing, University of Manchester.

White, R. (1985) Political regulators in British nursing. In: R. White (ed) *Political issues in nursing Volume 1,* J. Wiley and Sons, Chichester.

Whyte, L. (1985) Safe as houses? *Nursing Times, June 25, 48.*

Wilson-Barnett, J. (1988) Lend me your ear, *Nursing Times, 84, 33, 51-52.*

Wirth, J. (1979) *John Dewey as Educator,* Robert Krieger, New York.

Woolf, V. 1961 (1942) *The Death of the Moth and Other Essays,* Penguin, Harmondsworth.

Wright, H. and Giddey, M. (eds) (1993) *Mental health nursing: from first principles to professional practice,* Chapman and Hall, London.

Index